Ann Burkhardt, MA, OTR/L
Jodi Carlson, MS, OTR/L
Editors

Complementary Therapies in Geriatric Practice: Selected Topics

Complementary Therapies in Geriatric Practice: Selected Topics has been co-published simultaneously as *Physical & Occupational Therapy in Geriatrics,* Volume 18, Number 4 2001.

Pre-publication
REVIEWS,
COMMENTARIES,

" A SMORGASBORD OF INFORMATION. . . . Intellectually stimulating without being pedantic. This reader had difficulty putting it down."

Henrietta Gunderud, MPA, OTR/L
Private Practice Occupational Therapist, Wappingers Falls, New York

The Haworth Press, Inc.

Complementary Therapies in Geriatric Practice

Complementary Therapies in Geriatric Practice: Selected Topics has been co-published simultaneously as *Physical & Occupational Therapy in Geriatrics,* Volume 18, Number 4 2001.

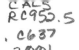
The *Physical & Occupational Therapy in Geriatrics* Monographic "Separates"

Below is a list of "separates," which in serials librarianship means a special issue simultaneously published as a special journal issue or double-issue *and* as a "separate" hardbound monograph. (This is a format which we also call a "DocuSerial.")

"Separates" are published because specialized libraries or professionals may wish to purchase a specific thematic issue by itself in a format which can be separately cataloged and shelved, as opposed to purchasing the journal on an on-going basis. Faculty members may also more easily consider a "separate" for classroom adoption.

"Separates" are carefully classified separately with the major book jobbers so that the journal tie-in can be noted on new book order slips to avoid duplicate purchasing.

You may wish to visit Haworth's website at . . .

http://www.HaworthPress.com

. . . to search our online catalog for complete tables of contents of these separates and related publications.

You may also call 1-800-HAWORTH (outside US/Canada: 607-722-5857), or Fax 1-800-895-0582 (outside US/Canada: 607-771-0012), or e-mail at:

getinfo@haworthpressinc.com

Complementary Therapies in Geriatric Practice: Selected Topics, edited by Ann Burkhardt, MA, OTR/L, FAOTA, BCN, and Jodi Carlson, MS, OTR/L (Vol. 18, No. 4, 2001). *"Dynamic. . . . Leads the reader through the current challenge of dealing with managed care, market-driven reforms, and the decreasing societal access to therapy. The book discusses the history of major foundations principles (energy medicine, naturopathic medicine assessment and diagnosis), healing by intention, bodywork therapies, mind-body therapies, and beginning/end life therapies." (Beth Ann Kneisley, MOT, OTR/L, Chairman, Occupational Therapy Assistant Program, Owens Community College, Toledo, Ohio)*

Aging and Developmental Disability: Current Research, Programming, and Practice Implications, edited by Joy Hammel, PhD, OTR/L, FAOTA, and Susan M. Nochajski, PhD, OTR (Vol. 18, No. 1, 2000). *Discusses the effectiveness of specific interventions targeted toward aging adults with developmental disabilities such as Down's Syndrome, cerebral palsy, autism, and epilepsy.*

Teaching Students Geriatric Research, edited by Margaret A. Perkinson, PhD, and Kathryn L. Braun, DrPH (Vol. 17, No. 2, 2000). *"An excellent collection of well-written papers. . . . The presentation of each model is intriguing and will entice instructors to think about how they may enhance their approaches to working with graduate students in both classroom situations and as research assistants." (Karen A. Roberto, PhD, Professor and Director, Center for Gerontology, Virginia Polytechnic Institute and State University, Blacksburg, Virginia)*

Aging in Place: Designing, Adapting, and Enhancing the Home Environment, edited by Ellen D. Taira, OTR/L, MPH, and Jodi L. Carlson, MS, OTR/L (Vol. 16, No. 3/4, 1999). *This important book examines the current trends in adaptive home designs for older adults and explores innovative home designs and studies for creating environments that offer optimal living for aging adults.*

The Mentally Impaired Elderly: Strategies and Interventions to Maintain Function, edited by Ellen D. Taira, OTR/L, MPH (Vol. 9, No. 3/4, 1991). *"Caregivers will benefit from this book as it provides information on methods and strategies to deal with mentally impaired elderly patients." (Senior News)*

Aging in the Designed Environment, edited by Margaret A. Christenson, MPH, OTR (Vol. 8, No. 3/4, 1990). *"Presents the environment as the untapped treatment modality that can maximize a person's functional abilities when designed effectively . . . integrates theory with practice to provide a very coherent and stimulating book." (Canadian Journal of Occupational Therapy)*

Successful Models of Community Long Term Care Services for the Elderly, edited by Eloise H. P. Killeffer, EdM, and Ruth Bennett, PhD (Vol. 8, No. 1/2, 1990). *"Provides invaluable information to practitioners, educators, policymakers, and researchers concerned with meeting the myriad needs of the elderly." (Patricia A. Miller, MEd, OTR, FAOTA, Assistant Professor of Clinical Occupational Therapy and Public Health, Columbia University)*

Assessing the Driving Ability of the Elderly: A Preliminary Investigation, edited by Ellen D. Taira, OTR/L, MPH (Vol. 7, No. 1/2, 1989). " 'The' *resource for older driver assessment. This new book provides a review of older driver literature, guidelines for practitioners who must assess older driver skills, and offers twenty-one screening instruments that test the visual, motor, and cognitive abilities of mature drivers." (Resources in Aging)*

Promoting Quality Long Term Care for Older Persons, edited by Ellen D. Taira, OTR/L, MPH (Vol. 6, No. 3/4, 1989). *Exciting programs in long term care–designed to better serve elderly persons with chronic diseases–are highlighted in this rich volume.*

Rehabilitation Interventions for the Institutionalized Elderly, edited by Ellen D. Taira, OTR/L, MPH (Vol. 6, No. 2, 1989). *"A sample of rehabilitation interventions which, combined in this volume, provide a holistic approach to gerontic services for those who are institutionalized." (Advances for Occupational Therapists)*

Community Programs for the Health Impaired Elderly, edited by Ellen D. Taira, OTR/L, MPH (Vol. 6, No. 1, 1989). *"This is an easy-to-read reference book occupational therapists can use to explore and develop techniques and programs to meet individual and community needs." (American Journal of Occupational Therapists)*

Community Programs for the Depressed Elderly: A Rehabilitation Approach, edited by Ellen D. Taira, OTR/L, MPH (Vol. 5, No. 1, 1987). *"A timely publication as recognition of the serious magnitude of depression amongst the elderly continues to grow." (Canadian Journal of Occupational Therapy)*

Therapeutic Interventions for the Person with Dementia, edited by Ellen D. Taira, OTR/L, MPH (Vol. 4, No. 3, 1986). *"Packed with useful information. The reader gains a better grasp of the patience, understanding, and flexibility needed to help these people. This is excellent reading for therapists and students and a valuable addition to the library of anyone working with the elderly." (American Journal of Occupational Therapy)*

Handbook of Innovative Programs for the Impaired Elderly, edited by Eloise H. P. Killeffer, EdM, Ruth Bennett, PhD, and Gerta Gruen, MPH (Vol. 3, No. 3, 1985). *"A handy source of ideas for promoting maintenance of physical abilities, restoring physical and mental abilities, and linking residents with organizations and services in the surrounding community and opening the long-term care facility to the community." (Canadian Journal of Occupational Therapy)*

A Handbook of Assistive Devices for the Handicapped Elderly: New Help for Independent Living, by Joseph M. Breuer, MA, RPT (Vol. 1, No. 2, 1982). *"Practical advice is coupled with a significant theoretical background and valuable experience." (Journal of the American Geriatrics Society)*

Complementary Therapies in Geriatric Practice: Selected Topics

Ann Burkhardt, MA, OTR/L, FAOTA, BCN
Jodi Carlson, MS, OTR/L
Editors

Complementary Therapies in Geriatric Practice: Selected Topics has been co-published simultaneously as *Physical & Occupational Therapy in Geriatrics*, Volume 18, Number 4 2001.

The Haworth Press, Inc.
New York • London • Oxford

Complementary Therapies in Geriatric Practice: Selected Topics has been co-published simultaneously as *Physical & Occupational Therapy in Geriatrics*, Volume 18, Number 4 2001.

The development, preparation, and publication of this work has been undertaken with great care. However, the publisher, employees, editors, and agents of The Haworth Press and all imprints of The Haworth Press, Inc., including The Haworth Medical Press® and The Pharmaceutical Products Press®, are not responsible for any errors contained herein or for consequences that may ensue from use of materials or information contained in this work. Opinions expressed by the author(s) are not necessarily those of The Haworth Press, Inc.

Cover design by Jennifer M. Gaska

Library of Congress Cataloging-in-Publication Data

Complementary therapies in geriatric practice : selected topics / Ann Burkhardt, Jodi Carlson, editors.
    p. cm.
    "Co-published simultaneously as Physical & occupational therapy in geriatrics, volume 18, number 4 2001."
    Includes bibliographical references and index.
    ISBN 0-7890-1431-9 (alk. paper) – ISBN 0-7890-1432-7 (alk. paper)
    1. Aged–Diseases–Alternative treatment. 2. Aged–Diseases–Rehabilitation. I. Burkhardt, Ann. II. Carlson, Jodi L.

RC952.5 .C637 2001
618.97′06–dc21

2001039956

Indexing, Abstracting & Website/Internet Coverage

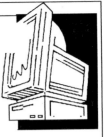

This section provides you with a list of major indexing & abstracting services. That is to say, each service began covering this periodical during the year noted in the right column. Most Websites which are listed below have indicated that they will either post, disseminate, compile, archive, cite or alert their own Website users with research-based content from this work. (This list is as current as the copyright date of this publication.)

(continued)

(continued)

Special Bibliographic Notes related to special journal issues
(separates) and indexing/abstracting:

- indexing/abstracting services in this list will also cover material in any "separate" that is co-published simultaneously with Haworth's special thematic journal issue or DocuSerial. Indexing/abstracting usually covers material at the article/chapter level.
- monographic co-editions are intended for either non-subscribers or libraries which intend to purchase a second copy for their circulating collections.
- monographic co-editions are reported to all jobbers/wholesalers/approval plans. The source journal is listed as the "series" to assist the prevention of duplicate purchasing in the same manner utilized for books-in-series.
- to facilitate user/access services all indexing/abstracting services are encouraged to utilize the co-indexing entry note indicated at the bottom of the first page of each article/chapter/contribution.
- this is intended to assist a library user of any reference tool (whether print, electronic, online, or CD-ROM) to locate the monographic version if the library has purchased this version but not a subscription to the source journal.
- individual articles/chapters in any Haworth publication are also available through the Haworth Document Delivery Service (HDDS).

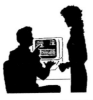

Complementary Therapies in Geriatric Practice: Selected Topics

CONTENTS

ABOUT THE EDITORS

Ann Burkhardt, MA, OTR/L, FAOTA, BCN, is Director of Occupational Therapy in the Department of Rehab Medicine at the New York Presbyterian Hospital, Columbia Presbyterian Center, New York, She also serves as Associate Professor of Clinical Occupational Therapy at Columbia University, as Professional Associate at Mercy College, and as Adjunct Professor at York College (CUNY). She is a Past President of the New York State Occupational Therapy Association. She is co-author of two texts: *Stroke Rehabilitation: A Function-Based Approach* and *A Therapist's Guide to Oncology: Medical Issues Affecting Management*, and was a columnist on the topic of CAM for *OT Week*, the national weekly publication of the American Occupational Therapy Association.

Jodi Carlson, MS, OTR/L, is a private practitioner in Westchester and Putnam Counties, New York. She works in adult group homes for the developmentally disabled, for Westchester and Putnam Hospice, and participates in research on developing occupational therapy programs for community settings. Ms. Carlson has practiced as an occupational therapist for six years. For four years she served as a home care occupational therapist of the Schizophrenia Research Unit of the New York State Psychiatric Institute.

Acknowledgments

The Guest Editors would like to thank the following people for serving as Adjunct Editorial Board Members in reviewing manuscripts for this text: Catherine Duffy, OTR/L, BCN, Advanced Clinician, Inpatient Rehabilitation, New York Presbyterian Hospital–Columbia Presbyterian; Linda Wong Ng, MA, OTR/L, Parker Jewish Geriatric Center; and Jane Sorensen, Private Practice, New York, NY.

Introduction

Ann Burkhardt, MA, OTR/L, FAOTA, BCN

As therapists move beyond the boundaries of traditional rehabilitation and medical model practice to wellness, they are expanding their practice skills to include complementary approaches. Rehabilitation and the complementary medicine movement are intrinsically compatible since they both tend to view people holistically–as more than merely the sum of component parts. Each philosophy emphasizes quality of life and empowers people to participate in life change and health enhancement.

In rehabilitation treatment, practitioners must address more with their clients than solely the complementary approach. The technique is rather a precursor or adjunct to components of a balanced lifestyle that relies upon the performance of tasks such as self-care, work, play, leisure, and rest (Kinney, Burkhardt, Mills, Swarbrick, & Sheinholtz, 1998). For involvement of a complementary technique to be considered treatment, rehabilitation theories must be the basis for intervention. Practice must be ethics-centered, with an appropriate rationale for therapy in which services provided enhance the individual's ability to assume or resume life roles with meaning and purpose.

Therapists who use these techniques will have studied to gain competency in the techniques prior to using the technique directly with clients. Therapists who are not competent in the activity may coach clients with whom they are working through the process of choosing classes

Ann Burkhardt is Director of Occupational Therapy, New York Presbyterian Hospital, Columbia–Presbyterian Medical Center, New York, NY.

[Haworth co-indexing entry note]: "Introduction." Burkhardt, Ann. Co-published simultaneously in *Physical & Occupational Therapy in Geriatrics* (The Haworth Press, Inc.) Vol. 18, Number 4, 2001, pp. 1-2; and: *Complementary Therapies in Geriatric Practice: Selected Topics* (ed: Ann Burkhardt, and Jodi Carlson) The Haworth Press, Inc., 2001, pp. 1-2. Single or multiple copies of this article are available for a fee from The Haworth Document Delivery Service [1-800-342-9678, 9:00 a.m. - 5:00 p.m. (EST). E-mail address: getinfo@haworthpressinc.com].

and a learning environment appropriate for their learning ability and personal style (Burkhardt & Parker, 1998).

Complementary techniques can often calm or focus a person before a therapist utilizes participation in activities and selected tasks. Many complementary techniques can direct people toward wellness behaviors, such as managing stress or increasing activity level. Some complementary techniques currently being utilized by therapists include guided imagery, manual therapies (such as massage, myofascial release, and craniosacral therapy), traditional Chinese movement or energy therapies (e.g., T'ai Chi C'huan and Qi Gong), aromatherapy, therapeutic touch, Reiki, neurolinguistic programming (NLP), meditation, yoga, music therapy, dance therapy, and traditional medicines such as Tibetan or Native American medicine, or other indigenous spiritualities (AOTA, 1998).

This volume describes several topics in complementary care which are important in geriatric rehabilitation. Therapist involvement in spirituality is of growing interest, and this topic reaches across all boundaries of complementary care. Mental Rehearsal, Tai Chi Chuan, and Energy Therapies are all examples of specific modalities or methods which can be used to enhance outcomes in rehabilitation treatment. And, finally, Well Elderly approaches to treatment are useful both in rehabilitation and prevention of the problems of aging. By providing information about these topics, we hope to expand possibilities in geriatric rehabilitation and prevention to enhance patient outcomes.

REFERENCES

Burkhardt, A., & Parker, J. (1998). OT Week, November 12, 1998, AOTA, Bethesda, MD, p. 11.

Complementary Care Survey Results. (1998). OT Week, November 26, 1998, AOTA, Bethesda, MD, p. 4.

Kinney, A., Burkhardt, A., Mills, J., Swarbrick, P., & Sheinholtz, M. (1998). Report of the Balanced Lifestyle Guide Taskforce, AOTA, Bethesda, MD.

Occupational Therapy as a Means to Wellness with the Elderly

Anne Hiller Scott, PhD, OTR, FAOTA
Danielle N. Butin, MPH, OTR
Diane Tewfik, MA, OTR
Ann Burkhardt, MA, OTR/L, BCN
Deborah Mandel, MA, OTR
Laurie Nelson, MA, OTR

SUMMARY. Therapists, as experts in promoting independence, have a role in providing wellness and health promotion programs in the community. This article features several models targeting the needs of the elderly, incorporating comprehensive functional wellness and prevention programs by occupational therapists. Oxford's Health Plans, Health Promotion, and Wellness department, under the direction of an occupational

Anne Hiller Scott is Director, Division of Occupational Therapy, Long Island University, 1 University Plaza, Brooklyn, NY 11201. Danielle N. Butin is Oxford Health Plans Manager, Health Promotion and Wellness, 44 South Broadway, White Plains, NY 10610-4419. Diane Tewfik is Associate Professor, Occupational Therapy, York College, Health Science Department, 94-20 Guy Brewer Blvd., Jamaica, NY 11451. Ann Burkhardt is Director of Occupational Therapy, New York Presbyterian Hospital, Columbia-Presbyterian Medical Center; Associate Clinical Professor, Programs in Occupational Therapy, Columbia University; and Clinical Associate, Mercy College, Dobbs Ferry, NY. Deborah Mandel is affiliated with the University of Southern California, Department of Occupational Science and Occupational Therapy, Clinical Instructor of Occupational Therapy, 1540 Alcazar CHP-133, Los Angeles, CA 90033. Laurie Nelson is affiliated with the California State University, Dominguez Hills, Occupational Therapy Department, Academic Fieldwork Coordinator, 1000 East Victoria Street, Carson, CA 90747.

[Haworth co-indexing entry note]: "Occupational Therapy as a Means to Wellness with the Elderly." Scott et al. Co-published simultaneously in *Physical & Occupational Therapy in Geriatrics* (The Haworth Press, Inc.) Vol. 18, Number 4, 2001, pp. 3-22 and: *Complementary Therapies in Geriatric Practice: Selected Topics* (ed: Ann Burkhardt and Jodi Carlson) The Haworth Press, Inc., 2001, pp. 3-22. Single or multiple copies of this article are available for a fee from The Haworth Document Delivery Service [1-800-342-9678, 9:00 a.m. - 5:00 p.m. (EST). E-mail address: getinfo@haworthpressinc.com].

3

therapist, has offered cost-effective programs, including health and nutrition screening, fall prevention, diabetes management, a sleep well/feel well educational series, and a member led walking club. The lifestyle redesign program emerging from the model of occupational science is presented. Research outcomes for a randomized controlled trial demonstrated significant benefits in a variety of health, function and quality of life domains based on the occupational therapy intervention with community based, culturally diverse well-elders. Lastly, the use of T'ai Chi in the ROM (Range of Motion) Dance program reviews the health benefits of T'ai Chi and resources available to implement this approach. Each of these programs serves as an evidence-based model for community-based practice. Implications for addressing public health goals articulated in Healthy People 2010 are also discussed. *[Article copies available for a fee from The Haworth Document Delivery Service: 1-800-342-9678. E-mail address: <getinfo@haworthpressinc.com> Website: <http://www.HaworthPress.com> © 2001 by The Haworth Press, Inc. All rights reserved.]*

KEYWORDS. Prevention, ROM dance, well elderly, occupational therapy, public health

With the advent of managed care and market driven reforms, occupational therapists, like other health care professionals, are striving to maintain and redefine their unique contributions to the field. Practitioners need to constantly justify efficacy in order to survive managed competition. McCormack (1997) has observed that in response to managed care, occupational therapy has developed a "functional outcome approach" with new opportunities emerging for practice. How practitioners accomplish this functional outcome approach in our everyday practice is crucial for ourselves as clinicians, as well as for the clients we serve. We must refine and develop a functional outcome approach to verify our efficacy to the managed care industry as well as for our own survival as a profession. Such practice trends have long been implemented in Canada, the United Kingdom, and Australia, where occupational therapists are an integral partner in implementation of health-based program initiatives for specific and targeted populations (Wilcox, 1998). A related development is evidence-based practice, which challenges practitioners to use therapeutic practices that demonstrate a solid track record with similar populations.

This article highlights several models targeting the needs of the elderly and incorporating comprehensive functional wellness and prevention programs. Occupational therapists can easily access outcomes to support the efficacy of practice using the models described here. The first was initiated as part of an HMO's (Oxford) Health Promotion and Wellness Department administered by an occupational therapist (Butin & Montgomery, 1997). The second is a comprehensive lifestyle redesign program formulated for the well elderly (Mandel, Jackson, Zemke, Nelson, & Clark, 1999) which emerged from research on "Occupational Therapy for Independent-Living Older Adults" (Clark, Azen, Zemke, Jackson, Carlson, Mandel, Hay, Josephson, Cherry, Hessel, Palmer, & Lipson, 1997). A third approach illustrates the therapeutic and health promotion benefits of complementary techniques, as documented in the research on ROM Dance (Tse & Bailey, 1992; Van Deusen & Harlow, 1987), which employs the ancient arts of T'ai Chi and meditation set to music as a vehicle to enhance postural alignment, reduce pain, and improve range of motion, mobility, balance, and diaphragmatic breathing. This program, which has existed for decades, demonstrates how occupational therapists can better serve our populations by integrating specific complementary tools within the framework of functional outcomes.

All therapists need to be aware of the major public health initiative, Healthy People 2010 (U. S. Dept., 2000). The goals of Healthy People 2010 are targeted for (1) increasing quality of life and achieving a longer healthier life and, (2) eliminating health disparities that may occur based on gender, race or ethnicity, disability, sexual orientation, education or income, and living in urban or rural locales. Each of the following programs provides opportunities to support some of the health promotion goals included in Healthy People 2010.

Each of the presented approaches clearly illustrates wellness programs designed for seniors that demonstrate not only quality care but also quality outcomes, the gold standard in a climate where evidence-based practice is becoming the bottom line. As evidence-based practice becomes the norm for practice, these programs offer successful prototypes. With the reemergence of community based practice, clinicians, educators, and students may employ these and related group-based interventions to verify functional outcomes for the elderly (Scott, 1999).

Wellness and health promotion form a viable frontier where tools such as education about behaviors and lifestyles are implemented for health maintenance, allowing consumers to assume responsibility for their own health (Butin & Montgomery, 1997). From the occupational therapy perspective, a state of health includes a balance of one's productive activity, emotional expression, social support, and positive interactions with the environment (Swarbrick, 1996). This definition draws from the core belief that occupation–the valued activities and fabric of everyday routine–provides meaning in life through engaging mind, body, and spirit. The following model programs demonstrate that occupational therapists, as experts in promoting functional independence, have a role in providing wellness and health promotion programs in the community and point to roles different therapists can assume in such programs.

HEALTH PROMOTION AND WELLNESS PROGRAMS AT OXFORD HEALTH PLANS

Oxford Health Plans, a health maintenance organization in the metropolitan New York area, offers highly innovative health programs for its Medicare population. The Medicare Health Promotion and Wellness Department, managed by an occupational therapist, Danielle N. Butin, MPH, OTR, develops and implements comprehensive wellness and health oriented programs for Medicare members. The goals of the department are to improve overall health and function of Medicare members and to decrease unnecessary health care utilization. Programs are designed to empower members with the information they need to make lifestyle changes (Butin & Montgomery, 1997). The occupational therapy manager also serves as a member of the HMO Workgroup on Care Management developed out of the Robert Wood Johnson Foundation Chronic Care Initiatives in HMO's project, headquartered at the American Association of Health Plans (AAHP) Foundation. As a member of the work group, the manager has been able to contribute an occupational therapy perspective to health promotion and program guidelines for managed care organizations (Boult, Paulwan, Fox, & Pacala, 1998). An account of how Oxford applied the findings of the workgroup to enhance its care management of the Medicare population is available (Butin, 1999).

The manager of the Health Promotion Department has designed and implemented innovative demonstration programs which have documented functional outcomes and cost-effectiveness. Prior to the development of a new program, the department's staff review health-related literature and meet with leading experts in the field to determine the best strategy for meeting the targeted needs of the Medicare members. The

Medicare Health Promotion Department has developed a number of major initiatives for health screening and management, including: (1) health risk screening and interventions; (2) nutrition screening and intervention; (3) fall prevention; (4) self-management courses and books for diabetes and COPD; (5) healthy aging seminars of "Oxford College" and, (6) a walking club (Butin & Montgomery, 1997). These programs provide members with the opportunity to process attitudes, information, and practice behaviors that promote healthy aging. By focusing on the behaviors, skills and strategies necessary to manage one's daily life, health-related changes occur. This framework is consistent with the basic tenets of occupational therapy.

Health Risk Screening and Intervention Program

The Health Risk Screening Intervention Program for Medicare members complies with the Health Care Financing Agency's (HCFA) Medicare Plus Choice regulations which require providing an initial assessment of all new enrollees' health care needs and assessing and treating enrollees with complex and serious medical conditions (HMO Workgroup on Care Management, 1999). The goal of this program is to identify members' risk levels early in order to achieve better patient management. By offering this service, Oxford can readily determine members' immediate needs and initiate an effective network of individualized services.

The Health Risk Screen, a standardized screening instrument, is administered through a telephone interview. The screen identifies members at low, moderate, and high risk for hospitalization. Members at high risk for hospitalization are automatically directed to geriatric case management. The geriatric case management team identifies, educates, and manages members at high risk for becoming ill. Members identified as moderate risk are sent to the Education and Outreach Department for individual assessment. This department is composed of associates who are skilled at listening to and understanding the complex needs of the elderly. They link members to community resources and social services. Members receive assistance with such issues as loss of a spouse, depression, isolation and the need for transportation.

A model for assessing function has been implemented as well. The assessment includes standardized ADL (Katz, Moskowitz, Jackson, & Jaffee, 1963) and IADL checklists (Lawton & Brody, 1969). It is computerized and administered during a telephone interview by Education and Outreach associates. The assessment identifies functional limitations that a member may experience. Limitations are addressed through the provision of resources and coordination of care with Geriatric Care Management nurses. For example, if a member with arthritis described meal preparation as painful, the associate would help the member to access meals on wheels or other food support programs. If this member had multiple functional limitations, then the associate would refer him/her to geriatric care management and they might recommend an occupational therapy evaluation to establish a plan of care to promote function and decrease pain.

Nutrition Screening and Intervention Program

The Nutrition Screening Intervention Program was developed as a means to prevent or reduce the significant health risks encountered by Medicare members suffering from malnutrition. By identifying members at risk and providing appropriate intervention and referral to community resources, nutrition issues can be effectively addressed, and cost benefits analyzed. Originally, Oxford Medicare Members were sent the Determine Checklist, a 10-item self-report scale developed by the Nutrition Screening Initiative. The tool screens for malnutrition indicators, such as financial difficulties, physiological challenges, psychological barriers, or educational deficiencies. Once areas of concern are identified, various interventions are initiated by the Education and Outreach team, such as referrals to dietitians, social workers, congregate meal sites, or transportation. Survey results are sent to the member's physician and social service agencies. This program was developed in conjunction with the Ross Products Division of Abbott Laboratories, which provided financial and physician education support.

During the pilot stage, the Nutrition Screening checklist was mailed to thousands of members residing in Brooklyn, New York. The mailing resulted in a 36-45% response rate. Training and outreach services were implemented and cognitive behavioral strategies were used to overcome resistance to the interventions. Subsequently, a telephone survey was instituted to reach more members and to increase the consistency of correctly recorded responses. Currently, Oxford incorporates the Nutrition Screen into the new member Health Risk Screening process. An attempt is made to offer all newly enrolled members a Nutrition Screen. From the sample of 1,116 Oxford members residing in Brooklyn, 482 high-risk members who received intervention assistance were compared with a control group of 634 high-risk members who refused intervention or could not be contacted. Importantly, utilization was evenly matched for both groups six months prior to the intervention phase. A review of pre- and post-claims data, including an evaluation of primary care physician visits, emergency room visits, individual practitioner visits, and hospital room and board costs, indicated that the program achieved an annual $300 savings per member. Future detailed analysis of members at risk in other locales is planned.

Fall Prevention Program

Building on the research findings of Tinetti, Baker, Garrett, Gottshalk, Koch, and Horowitz (1993), the Fall Prevention Program aims to reduce the rate of injurious falls among program participants. Each fall can cost up to $15,000 in medical expenses. Oxford is collaborating with Dr. Tinetti and her team at Yale University to implement and evaluate a Fall Prevention model with a larger sample and a wider range of interventions.

Occupational therapists will be responsible for functional adaptations (e.g., environmental adaptations, compensatory strategies, and adaptive equipment), while physical therapists will facilitate improvement in physical aspects of functioning (e.g., balance, range of motion, and strength). The program will reach out to members age 70 and older in two boroughs of New York City. The program evaluation will assess the effectiveness of the multi-factorial risk abatement program in decreasing the incidence of injurious falls. The projected sample of this Fall Prevention model is approximately 2000 members randomized into a control and an intervention group. A two-part telephone screening process will be administered to identify those members who are at high risk for falling. Their contributing factors are assessed during baseline evaluations by physical and occupational therapists. Then risk reduction protocols will be initiated to address the identified risk factors. Some of the areas that will be addressed include training for gait, balance, range of motion, environmental modifications to improve home safety, and nursing visits for postural hypotension and utilization of multiple medications. In addition, participants may receive recommendations on safe footwear, bathroom transfers, and activities of daily living. Finally, existing services within a member's benefit plan are utilized to address poor nutritional status, vision and hearing deficits, foot problems, and depression.

Options for Living with Diabetes Program:
A Course in Self-Management

The Options for Living with Diabetes Program, based on Lorig's research (Lorig & Holman, 1989; Lorig, Seleznick, Lubeck, Ung, Chastian, &

Holman, 1989) is another successful program offered through the Health Prevention and Wellness Department. This program is a 7-week, 3-hour a week self-management series developed to educate members about diabetes. It is designed to teach functional skills and knowledge needed to self-manage a chronic condition. Health professionals present topics pertinent to living with diabetes, including understanding the condition, nutrition, exercise, medications and complications, coping skills, functional daily living skills, and wellness. A similar program has also been developed for chronic obstructive pulmonary disease. Comprehensive self-help books written by an interdisciplinary group of experts are available to members as reference guides to reinforce workshop sessions.

Members attending the Options for Living with Diabetes Program are invited to attend monthly support groups after the completion of the program. To assist investigators in evaluating outcomes of the program, all participants complete the SF-12, a self-report instrument on physical and mental functioning (Ware, Kosinski, & Keller, 1996), along with Measures of Illness Intrusiveness (Devins, Binik, Hutchinson, Hollomby, Barre, & Gutterman, 1983) and Self-Efficacy to Manage Chronic Conditions (Lorig, Stewart, Ritter, Gonzalez, Laurent, & Lynch, 1996). Preliminary results from a sample of 109 members throughout the boroughs of New York, demonstrated a utilization savings of approximately $100 per member/per month for those who participated in the program. Additional pre-program vs. post-program cost comparisons are planned.

Oxford College Health Education Series

Another promising program series is the "Oxford College" Health Education Seminar. The Health Promotion department has worked with multi-disciplinary experts in the field of aging to develop curricula and health education materials that are practical and easy to understand. Lectures presented by health professionals target the interests and needs of older adults. Past seminars have included Healthy Eating, Focusing on Fats and Cholesterol, Getting Healthy Through Physical Activity, Sleep Well–Feel Well, and Managing Medications. Recently a series of seminars on Complementary Care was implemented, including Energy Work, Nutritional Supplements, and Herbal Remedies. Interestingly, these complementary care seminars have been filled to capacity. Guidelines and suggestions are made for practical solutions to health problems.

In a 3-month analysis of feedback from members who attended the Sleep Well–Feel Well lecture series, 96% reported that they had a greater understanding of sleep and how it affects their health, and 61%

reported using the sleep journals provided as an aid to recognize non-productive sleep habits. Another successful feature of the program was a relaxation tape, which 77% reported using. The tape was developed by an occupational therapist, Judith Parker, who is affiliated with a complementary care practice (Parker, 1997). These types of programs can substantially contribute to membership satisfaction and retention (Schauffer & Rodriguez, 1994).

Walking Club

Finally, the Walking Club is another example of the Healthy Aging Program. The club is supported by the Health Promotion and Wellness Department and managed by members. Member leaders choose to serve as "coaches" and organize walk times and sites. To date, 28 clubs are in existence with 739 members. The clubs meet 2-3 times each week for approximately 2 hours. Members walk on outdoor trails, tracks, and in malls. A Manhattan club walks around the reservoir in Central Park. The Walking Club is an opportunity for older adults to walk together while building social ties, an essential component of maintaining one's health (Baldassare, Rosenfield, & Rook, 1984).

Summary

Butin and Montgomery have stated that occupational therapists, as "experts in functional analysis and rehabilitation, have a role to play in the design and implementation of programs that enhance the confidence and function of older adults" (1997, p. 3). By finding the best way to teach functional strategies, the occupational therapist can empower older adults to incorporate behaviors that translate into prevention or management of chronic conditions. Managed care can be a natural partner for occupational therapists. Cost benefits can be achieved by using a "functional outcomes approach" and by expanding occupational therapists' knowledge to incorporate the principles of wellness and health promotion.

OCCUPATIONAL THERAPY FOR INDEPENDENT-LIVING OLDER ADULTS: UNIVERSITY OF SOUTHERN CALIFORNIA'S WELL ELDERLY STUDY

The role of occupational therapy interventions in promoting health, quality of life, and in enhancing engagement in more active and satisfying lifestyles has been demonstrated in the University of Southern California's Well Elderly Study (Clark, Azen, Zemke, Jackson, Carlson, Mandel, Hay, Josephson, Cherry, Hessel, Palmer, & Lipson, 1997). The research, "Occupational Therapy for Independent-Living Older Adults: A Randomized Controlled Trial," documents the preventive impact of occupational therapy with a population that included 361 elders living independently in subsidized housing in the Los Angeles area. The ethnic composition of the population was 11% Hispanic, 17% African American, 23% White, and 47% Asian. Baseline evaluations included medical history, physical examination, administration of the Tinetti Balance Examination (Tinetti, 1986), Mini Mental Status examination (MMSE) (Teng & Chui, 1987), the Geriatric Depression Scale (Yesavage, Brink, & Rose, 1983), and the LaRue Global Assessment (LaRue, Bank, Jarvik, & Hetland, 1979). Inclusion criteria required subjects to live independently, not exhibit marked dementia, and to score at least at the 75% level on all measures.

The research design included three randomized groups seen over the treatment period of 9 months. One group received occupational therapy (2 hours per week in group treatment and 9 hours of individual treatment over the course of the study). A second group, the social control group, was offered group activities such as games, dances, and craft projects provided by nonprofessionals for the same total amount of exposure as the occupational therapy group. The non-treatment control group received no intervention.

To assess program effectiveness, participants were evaluated on fifteen self-rated measures of vitality, physical and psychological health, and life satisfaction. Outcome measures were: Functional Status Questionnaire (Jette & Cleary, 1987), Life Satisfaction Index-Z (Burckhardt, 1985; Burckhardt, Woods, Schultz, & Ziebarth, 1989), Center for Epidemiologic Studies (CES) Depression Scale (Radloff, 1977), Medical Outcomes Study (MOS) Short Form General Health Survey (Stewart, Hays, & Ware, 1988), and the Rand 36-Item Health Status Survey, Short Form-36 (RAND SF-36) (Hays, Sherbourne, & Mazel, 1993; Ware & Sherbourne, 1992).

The occupational therapy treatment group displayed significant benefits across the majority of domains for health and quality of life, and experienced improvement, or fewer declines, on the outcome measures in comparison with the control group. Eleven outcome variables were significant compared to the social control group and 10 in contrast to the non-treatment control group.

OCCUPATIONAL THERAPY PROGRAM
USED IN THE WELL ELDERLY STUDY

The organizing premise of occupational therapy is the role of every-day activities or occupations in establishing routine and infusing meaning into daily life. The principles of occupational science were applied in the Lifestyle Redesign Program. Occupational science is defined as the "study of the form, function and meaning of occupation" (Clark, Wood, & Larson, 1993, p. 3). Occupations must be culturally relevant and personally meaningful to participants to potentially generate a transformative experience for the person within their environment and their sociocultural context (Carlson, Mandel, Zemke, & Clark, 1998).

Both individual and group treatments were designed to meet each participant's constellation of valued goals and activities. The occupational therapy treatment protocol for the Well Elderly Program Model consisted of (1) introduction to the power of occupations, (2) aging, health, and occupation, (3) transportation, (4) safety, (5) social relationships, (6) cultural awareness, (7) finances, and (8) integrative (Mandel et al., 1999). The focus of the intervention was to educate the participants about the impact of everyday occupations. This knowledge enables them to organize a healthy and meaningful pattern of activities and to deal with fears, which can perpetuate immobility and stagnation. In the context of a group setting structured by the protocol of the Well Elderly Program, the occupational therapist challenged participants to engage in occupations supporting personal goals for life-style redesign (Mandel, Jackson, Zemke, Nelson, & Clark, 1999).

CLARA: CASE ILLUSTRATION OF LIFESTYLE REDESIGN

For some elders, the physical and psychological losses of aging contribute to an ever-shrinking circle of community, social, and occupational participation. Valued occupations can be jettisoned in the process, contributing to mounting losses of treasured and life-sustaining occupations. We will briefly discuss Clara, who was 77 and lived alone in the Angelus Housing Plaza. She offers an example of the Lifestyle Redesign Program, and her case was documented in "The Well Elderly Study: Implementing Lifestyle Redesign" (Mandel, Jackson, Zemke, Nelson, & Clark, 1999, pp. 16-17).

With advancing age, obesity, diabetes, and mobility problems compounded by using a walker, Clara feared that she might fall and avoided using stairs. She ventured out to the familiar environs of the apartment complex and promenade to crochet and talk with her friends but otherwise curtailed community travel. For Clara, as for many frail elders, fear of falling was a powerful constraint.

Through ongoing participation in the program, Clara found support and encouragement from the occupational therapist and her group to participate in an outing to a farmer's market that was an hour away from the apartment complex. Although this created several challenges for her, she reluctantly committed to the field trip, which unexpectedly presented her with the need to confront her mobility fears both literally and figuratively. At the destination, she was assisted by the occupational therapist and her peers in not only negotiating a flight of stairs but also an escalator, something she had not done in a decade. As Clara tells it, "That day I did two things I thought I would never do. That night when I thought about it, I thought when people have faith in you, and they say you can do it–you can!" (Mandel, Jackson, Zemke, Nelson, & Clark, 1999, p. 17). This outing represented one small step for the group but a giant step for Clara.

But did this initial risk taking, under the supportive guidance of the occupational therapist and group, generate into further new horizons for Clara after the research study ended? Subsequently, Clara, with a small group of seniors in her project, decided to test their mettle in the LA marathon. The plan was for those using walkers to follow those racing in wheelchairs. Braving a steady drizzle, by 6:30 a.m. Clara had jockeyed her way through crowds of thousands awaiting her starting time. She was the only one of her group to actually follow up and do it. At the designated time "she waded into the edge of the throng and she was off. By the time Clara had walked a half a mile all of the other marathon participants were nowhere to be seen and the street sweepers were starting to clean up. Her friend held an umbrella over her head and wondered if Clara wanted to do more. Yes, she wanted to go on. Clara has a photo of herself, at the age of 77, standing with her walker, arms raised in victory, under the one mile marker of the race" (Mandel, Jackson, Zemke, Nelson, & Clark, 1999, p. 17).

Through her participation in the program, supported by the occupational therapist and fellow group members, Clara was able to reframe her view of her self and her potential. "She shifted from a person confined by limitations to one who discovered a new sense of freedom and opportunity for more meaningful occupations . . . she found the courage to accept new challenges and create a healthy more satisfying life" (Mandel, 4/6/1999, personal communication).

EAST MEETS WEST: THE ROM DANCE RELAXATION AND EXERCISE PROGRAM

The section that follows describes the effective use of several complementary modalities (T'ai Chi C'huan, meditation, visualization, and music) in a therapeutic intervention program known as ROM (Range of Motion) Dance. In a unique marriage of East and West, ROM Dance (Harlowe & Yu, 1984; Harlowe & Yu, 1997) represents a synthesis of the gentle motion of T'ai Chi C'huan, music, poetry, relaxation, and imagery. The ancient Chinese martial art of T'ai Chi C'huan, also known as shadow boxing, has been called a "kinder, gentler workout" (Shine, 1993) for those with arthritis and other conditions that require low impact activity.

There is a growing body of research documenting the health benefits of T'ai Chi with the elderly. Recent findings with elders report reduction and delayed onset of first or multiple falls and reduction in fear of falling (Wolf, Barnhart, Ellison, Coogler, & Horak, 1997); improved balance, sway, range of motion, decreased perceived pain, and lessened trait anxiety (Ross, Bohannon, Davis, & Gurchiek, 1999); increased balance and strength (Wolfson, Whipple, Derby, Judge, King, Amerman, Schmidt, & Smyers 1996); enhanced strength of knee extensor/flexor muscle groups, increased thoracic/lumbar flexibility and increased VO_2max (Lan, Lai, Chen, & Wong, 1998); reduced anxiety, depression, fatigue, and tension in persons with rheumatoid arthritis (Province, Hadley, & Hornbrook, 1995); and lowered blood pressure (Bankhead, 1998).

The ROM Dance Program is also part of the treatment protocol of the Well-Elderly study discussed above. The ROM Dance is a range of motion exercise and relaxation program developed in 1981, funded with a grant from the Wisconsin Chapter of the Arthritis Foundation (Harlowe & Yu, 1984). The authors are an occupational therapist, Diane Harlowe, MS, OTR, FAOTA, and Patricia Yu, MA, a health educator and certified T'ai Chi instructor with over 28 years of experience. The actual ROM Dance sequence lasts 7 minutes. Graceful, fluid range of motion exercises are accompanied by soothing refrains composed and performed by Ms. Yu, with an evocative text of poetry and rich images. It is multisensory, drawing the participant into a transformative mind-body experience.

There are three ROM Dance videos; the "ROM Dance in Sunlight" is performed in both seated and standing positions. "ROM Dance, Seated" is adapted for wheelchair use. A third, "ROM Dance in Moonlight," was created for people with lupus erythematosis who should avoid the sun. Six audiotapes include "Releasing Stress and Pain." In addition, "T'ai Chi Fundamentals, A Systematic Approach for Mastering T'ai-Chi" (1999) is a video for health professionals with analysis of clinical applications and physical benefits by Jill Johnson, MS, PT, GCS and Tricia Yu, MA. A companion video "T'ai Chi Fundamentals: Simplified Exercises for Beginners" (1999) is oriented to the general population from the professional athlete to those with physical limitations.

ROM Dance has been used for a variety of conditions and diagnoses, including chronic pain, arthritis, stroke, post-surgical trauma, back pain, and depression (Harlowe & Yu, 1997). It is performed both on a group or individual treatment basis in a variety of settings, including senior centers, hospice, home health, acute and long-term facilities. Support groups for individuals with HIV/AIDS, Parkinson's, chronic fatigue, lupus erythematosis, and fibromyalgia include this uplifting therapeutic routine in their programs (Harlowe & Yu, 1997).

To use ROM Dance therapeutically, a media kit and manual are available with detailed instructions for teaching the dance sequence and relaxation experience (Harlowe & Yu, 1984; Harlowe & Yu, 1997). The manual illustrates how to implement the seven principles of movement and relaxation: attention to the present, diaphragmatic breathing, postural alignment, awareness of movement, slow movement, relaxed movement, and imagination–all of which create a valuable prescription for renewal and integration of body, mind, and spirit. Workshops are offered for prospective instructors and certification is also an option.

ROM Dance has been featured in the "Encyclopedia of Body-Mind Disciplines" (Allison, 1999). An efficacy study (Van Deusen & Harlowe, 1987) with patients with rheumatoid arthritis using ROM Dance included control subjects who participated in traditional regimes of exercise and rest and the experimental group which used ROM Dance. Each group participated for eight weeks. On evaluation four months after the program, the ROM Dance participants demonstrated significantly greater range of motion in the upper extremities "although the reported frequency of exercise and rest was greater in the control group. Post program reports of enjoyment (of the exercise routine) were significantly higher for control than experimental subjects" (Van Deusen & Harlowe, 1987, p. 90).

PROMOTING HEALTH IN FUTURE PRACTICE

Occupational therapy as a profession is renewing its commitment to health promotion and wellness (Burkhardt, Kinney, Mills, Swarbrick & Scheinholtz, 1998; Swarbrick & Burkhardt, 1998). In concert with the awareness of the impact of lifestyle habits and patterns on health and illness (Lee & Estes, 1997), occupational therapists have traditionally worked with lifestyle issues of those experiencing disability and chronic illness. This population also has much to gain from a health promotion focus (Patrick, 1997; Teague, Cipriano & McGhee, 1990). Healthy People 2000 (U. S. Dept., 1990) suggests goals for those with disabilities, which are very resonant with the domain of occupational therapy: increase leisure and physical activity, decrease adverse health effects from stress, reduce secondary disability associated with spinal cord injury and traumatic brain injury and for those with chronic disabling conditions–provide patient education, community resources and self-help resources.

On the other hand, the more recently issued Healthy People 2010 (U. S. Dept., 2000), summons us to heed the leading health indicators: physical inactivity, overweight and obesity, tobacco use, substance abuse, responsible sexual behavior, mental illness, injury and violence, environmental quality, and access to health care. Physical inactivity is a major cause of morbidity and mortality in the elderly. People with physical disabilities are also less active than those without disabilities. Currently, 40% of adults engage in no leisure time physical activity, and obesity has doubled in the past two decades (U. S. Dept., 2000). By age 75, one in three men and one in two women engage in no regular physical leisure activity.

The common thread of each of these programs is the potential for community-based elders to engage in authentic occupational therapy empowering them through health promoting occupations. Each meets the challenge of targeting functional outcomes and provides a prototype for evidence-based practice. Consider how these programs meet the description of community health proposed in Healthy People 2010: "over the years, it has become clear that individual health is closely linked with community health–the health of the community and environment in which individuals live, work and play. Likewise, community health is profoundly affected by the collective behaviors, attitudes, and beliefs of everyone who lives in the community" (U.S. Dept., 2000, pp. 6-7).

Therapists need to think outside of the box and bring health promotion to traditional and nontraditional settings. Models are being developed to include occupational therapy students in wellness groups in community settings (Scott, 1999). An article entitled the "Top 10 emerging practice areas to watch in the new millennium: Where will you practice in 2010?" discusses opportunities for new markets in several areas that are relevant to the aging population, including private practice community health services, health and wellness consulting, driver rehabilitation and training, design and accessibility consulting and home modification, and low vision services (Johansson, 1999). The Commission for Accreditation for Rehabilitation Facilities (CARF) not only includes standards in traditional rehabilitation and industrial programs to address health promotion but has recently developed standards for agencies that offer wellness programs, which should provide a timely venue for innovative programming (New Standards, 1997). Some of the programmatic elements of each of these models could be applied in CARF accredited sites. The workplace is also a particularly important area of focus with OSHA's proposal for national ergonomic standards. As the workforce ages and more elders continue full or part-time employment, promoting their productivity will have many implications. As we begin this new century, occupational therapists should be poised to offer a full continuum of health promotion and wellness services to all people, wherever they may fall on the health-illness continuum: After all, wellness is for everyone! As therapists, let us promote in our practice the new vision statement of the American Occupational Therapy Association, to insure that "the contribution of occupational therapy to health, wellness, productivity and quality of life are widely used, understood and valued by society" (AOTA Tackles, 2000).

REFERENCES

Allison, N. (1999). *The Illustrated Encyclopedia of Body-Mind Disciplines*. Rosen Publishing Group, NY.

AOTA tackles strategic issues. (aota.org/nonmembers/area1/links/link107.asp). 2000, Nov. 3).

Baldassare, M., Rosenfield, N., & Rook, K. (1984). The types of social relationships predicting elderly well-being. *Research on Aging 6*, 549-559.

Bankhead, C. (1998). T'ai Chi helps lower BP in elderly showing benefit of light physical activity. *Medical Tribune for the Family Physician, April 16 (39)* 8, 10.

Boult, C., Paulwan, T. F., Fox, P. D., & Pacala, J. T. (1998). Identification and assessment of high-risk seniors. *American Journal of Managed Care, August 4* (8), 1137-1144.

Brummel-Smith, K. V. (1999). Geriatrics in managed care: Essential components of geriatric care provided through health maintenance organizations. *Journal of American Geriatric Society 46*, 303-308.

Burckhardt, C. S., Woods, S. L., Shultz, A. A., & Ziebarth, D. S. (1989). Quality of life of adults with chronic illness: A psychometric study. *Research in Nursing and Health 12*, 347-354.

Burckhardt, C. C. (1985). The impact of arthritis on quality of life. *Nursing Research, 34*, 11-16.

Burkhardt, A., Kinney, A., Mills, J., Swarbrick, P., & Scheinholtz, M. (1998, December). Balanced lifestyle concept paper. Balanced Lifestyle Task Force. Unpublished paper. AOTA.

Butin, D. (1999). A workshop on better care for seniors. *Healthplan Magazine*, Nov/Dec, 67-71. (RWJ Workgroup reference).

Butin, D. N., & Montgomery, A. (1997, September). Health promotion programs for older adults: The Oxford health plans model for innovative programming. American Occupational Therapy Association, *Gerontology Special Interest Section Quarterly 20*(3), 1-4.

Clark, F., Wood, W., & Larson, E. A. (1993). Occupational science: Occupational therapy's legacy for the 21st century. In M. E. Niestadt, & E. B. Crepau (Eds.), *Willard & Spackman's Occupational Therapy* (9th ed., pp. 13-20). Philadelphia/NY: Lippincott.

Clark, F., Azen, S. P., Zemke, R., Jackson, J., Carlson, M., Mandel, D., Hay, J., Josephson, K., Cherry, B., Hessel, C., Palmer, M. S., & Lipson, L. (1997). Occupational therapy for independent-living older adults. A randomized controlled trial. *Journal of the American Medical Society: Oct 22/29* (278) 16, 1321-1326.

Devins, G. M., Binik, Y. M., Hutchinson, T. A., Hollomby, D. J., Barre, P. E., & Guttman, R. D. (1983). The emotional impact of end-stage renal disease: Importance of patients' perceptions of intrusiveness and control. *International Journal of Psychiatric Medicine 13*, 327-343.

Edlin, M. (1998, Jan/Feb). Nutrition screening initiatives for seniors. *Health Plan*, 30-31.

Harlowe, D., & Yu, P. (1984). *The ROM Dance: A range of motion exercise and relaxation program.* Madison, WI: Uncharted Publishing Company:.

Harlowe, D., & Yu, P. (1997). *The ROM Dance: A range of motion exercise and relaxation program.* Madison, WI: Uncharted Publishing Company.

Hawranik, P. (1991). A clinical possibility: Prevention of health problems after the age of 65. *Journal of Gerontological Nursing 17*(11), 20-25.

Hays, R. D., Sherbourne, C. D., & Mazel, R. M. (1993). The RAND 36-item health survey 1.0. *Health Economy 2*, 217-227.

Healthy People 2000. (1990). Department of Health and Human Services. Washington, D.C: US Government Printing Office.

HMO Workgroup on Care Management. (1999). *Establishing relations with community resource organizations: An imperative for managed care organizations serving Medicare beneficiaries.* Washington, D.C.: AAHP Foundation.

Jackson, J., Carlson, M., Mandel, D., Zemke, R., & Clark, F. (1998). Occupation in lifestyle redesign: The well-elderly study occupational therapy program. *American Journal of Occupational Therapy 52*(5), 326-336.

Jette, A. M., & Cleary, P. D. (1987). Functional disability assessment. *Physical Therapy*, 67, 1854-1859.

Johansson, C. (1999). Top 10 emerging practice areas to watch in the new millennium: Where will you practice in 2010? *OT Week*, Jan. 17. (aota.org) Newsroom Menu.

Katz, S., Ford, A. B., Moskowitz, R. W., Jackson, B. A., & Jaffee, M. W. (1963). Studies of illness in the aged: The index of ADL: A standardized measure of biological and psychosocial function. *Journal of the American Medical Association 185*, 914-919.

Lan, C., Lai, J. S., Chen, S. Y., & Wong, M. K. (1998). 12 month Tai Chi training in the elderly: Its effects on health and fitness. *Medical Science and Sports Exercise, Mar 30*, 3, 345-351.

LaRue, A., Bank, L., Jarvik, L., & Hetland, M. (1979). Health in old age: How do physicians' ratings and self-ratings compare? *Journal of Gerontology 34*, 687-691.

Lawton, M. P., & Brody, E. M. (1969). Assessment of older people: Self-maintaining and instruments of activities of daily living, *The Gerontologist 9*(3), 179-186.

Lee, P., & Estes, C. (1997). *The nation's health.* (5th Edition). Jones and Bartlett.

Lorig, K., Stewart, A., Ritter, P., Gonzalez, V., Laurent, D., & Lynch, J. (1996). *Outcome measures for health education and other health care interventions.* Sage Publications.

Lorig, K., & Holman, H. (1989). Long-term outcomes of an arthritis self-management study: Effects of reinforcement efforts. *Social Sciences 29*(2), 221-224.

Lorig, K., Seleznick, M., Lubeck, D., Ung, Chastain, R. L., & Holman, H. R. (1989). Effects of a self-care education program on medical visits. *JAMA 250*(21), 2952-2956.

Mandel, D., Jackson, J., Zemke, R., Nelson, L., & Clark, F. (1999). *The well-elderly study: Implementing Lifestyle Redesign.* American Occupational Therapy Association: Bethesda, MD.

McCormack, G. (1997). What is nontraditional practice. *OT Practice* February, 2, 17-20.

New standards for accreditation. (1997). *OT WEEK*, p. 10, June 12.

Oxford Health Plans debuts medical nutrition therapy benefit. (1997). *ADA Courier* February, 36(2), 1.

Parker, J. (1997). Our role as growth facilitators. *OT Practice* February, 2, 20-21.

Patrick, D. (1997). Rethinking prevention for people with disabilities. *American Journal of Health Promotion* (March/April).

Province, M. A., Hadley E. C., Hornbrook, M. C. et al. (1995). The effects of exercise on falls in elderly patients. A preplanned meta-analysis of the FICSIT trails. Frailty and injuries: Cooperative studies of intervention techniques. *JAMA 273*, 1341-1347.

Radloff, L. (1977). The CES-D Scale: A self-report depression scale for research in general populations. *Applied Psychological Measurements 1*, 385-401.

Ross, M. C., Bohannon, A. S., Davis, D. C., & Gurchier, L. (1999). The effects of a short-term exercise program on movement, pain, and mood in the elderly: Results of a pilot study. *Journal of Holistic Nursing, June, 17* (2), 139-147.

Schauffler, H. H., & Rodriguez, P. (1994). Availability and utilization of health promotion programs and satisfaction with health plans. *Medical Care 32*, 1182-1190.

Scott, A. (1999). Wellness works: Community service health promotion groups led by occupational therapy students. *American Journal of Occupational Therapy 53*, 6, 566-574.

Shine, J. (1993). T'ai Chi: A kinder gentler workout. *Arthritis Today* January/February, 31-33.

Stewart, A. L., Hays, R. D., & Ware, J. E. (1988). The MOS Short-Form general health survey. *Medical Care 2*, 217-227.

Swarbrick, P. (1996). The Wellness Connection. *OT Week* September 12, 12-13.

Swarbrick, P., & Burkhardt, A. The role of occupational therapy in wellness promotion and disease prevention. Draft, June 12, 1998.

Tai Chi Fundamentals: A Systematic approach for Mastering Tai Chi. (1999). Videotape. Uncharted Country, PO Box 3332, Madison, WI 53704.

Teague, M. L., Cipriano, R. E., & McGhee, V. L. (1990). Health promotion as a rehabilitation service for people with disabilities. *Journal of Rehabilitation*, 52-56.

Teng, E., & Chui, H. (1987). The Modified Mini-Mental Status (3MS) Examination. *Journal of Clinical Psychiatry 48*, 314-317.

Tse, S., & Bailey, D. M. (1992). T'ai Chi and postural control in the well-elderly. *American Journal of Occupational Therapy 46* (4), 295-300.

Tinetti, M. E. (1986). Performance oriented assessment of mobility problems in elderly patients. *Journal of American Geriatric Society 34*, 119-126.

Tinetti, M. E., Baker, D. I., Garrett, P. A., Gottschalk, M., Koch, M. L., & Horowitz, R. I. (1993). Yale ficsit: Risk factor abatement strategy for fall prevention. *Journal of the American Geriatric Society, 4*, 315-320.

U.S. Department of Health and Human Services. (1988). *Proceedings of the Surgeon General's workshop: Health promotion and aging.* U.S. Government Printing Office: Washington, DC.

U.S. Department of Health and Human Services. *Healthy People 2010* (Conference Edition, in Two Volumes). U. S. Government Printing Office: Washington: D.C.

Van Deusen, J., & Harlowe, D. (1987). Efficacy of the ROM Dance program for adults with rheumatoid arthritis. *American Journal of Occupational Therapy 41*(2), 90-95.

Walker, S. (1992). Wellness for elders. *Holistic Nurse Practice 7*(1), 38-45.

Ware, J. E., Kosinski, M., & Keller, S. D. (1996). A 12-Item Short-Form Health Survey: Construction of scales and preliminary tests of reliability and validity. *Medical Care 34*(3), 220-233.

Ware, J. E., & Sherbourne, C. D. (1992). The MOS 36-home short form general health survey (SF-36). *Medical Care 30*, 478-481.

Wolf, S. L., Barnhart, H., Ellison, G. L., Coogler, C. E., & Horak, F. B. (1997). The effect of Tai Chi Quan and computerized balance training on postural stability in older subjects. *Physical Therapy 77*(4), 371-384.

Wolf, S. L., Barnhart, H. X., Kutner, N. G., McNeely, E., Coogler, C., & Xu, T. (1996). Reducing frailty and falls in older persons: An investigation of t'ai chi and computerized balance training. *Journal of American Geriatric Society 44* 599-600.

Wolfson, L., Whipple, R., Derby, C., Judge, J., King, M., Amerman, P., Schmidt, L., & Smyers, D. (1996). Balance and strength training in older adults: Intervention gains and t'ai chi maintenance. *Journal of American Geriatric Society 44*, 498-506.

Wood, V., Wylie, M. L., & Sheafor, B. (1969). An analysis of short self-reported measures of life satisfaction. *Journal of Gerontology 24*, 465-469.

Yesavage, J. A., Brink, T. L., Rose, T. L. et. al. (1983). Development and validation of a geriatric depression screening scale. *Journal of Psychiatric Residence 17*, 37-49.

Yu, T., Johnson, J., & Krapu, T. M. (1999). Research on t'ai chi c'huan. (http://members. aol.com/sltcca/research/

The Application of Tai Chi Chuan
in Rehabilitation and Preventive Care
of the Geriatric Population

Maureen McKenna, PhD, PT

SUMMARY. Falls in the elderly population are relatively common occurrences. Potential trauma as a result of these falls is more costly than the introduction of preventive approaches. One of these interventions is the use of Tai Chi Chuan. Regular practice of this form of exercise by the impaired and the well elderly produces important benefits, including a reduced risk of falls. The problems of the elderly, the physical aspects of Tai Chi, research information supporting the benefits of this form of exercise, and the history of its development are included in this overview. *[Article copies available for a fee from The Haworth Document Delivery Service: 1-800-342-9678. E-mail address: <getinfo@haworthpressinc.com> Website: <http://www.HaworthPress.com> © 2001 by The Haworth Press, Inc. All rights reserved.]*

KEYWORDS. Tai Chi, elderly, fall prevention

This article provides an overview of the historical background of Tai Chi, addresses some general problems of the elderly population, some

Maureen McKenna is a Licensed Physical Therapist and Licensed Marriage and Family Therapist in California. Her Current position is: Assistant Professor of Physical Therapy, Wheeling Jesuit University, 316 Washington Avenue, Wheeling, WV 26003.

[Haworth co-indexing entry note]: "The Application of Tai Chi Chuan in Rehabilitation and Preventive Care of the Geriatric Population." McKenna, Maureen. Co-published simultaneously in *Physical & Occupational Therapy in Geriatrics* (The Haworth Press, Inc.) Vol. 18, Number 4, 2001, pp. 23-34; and: *Complementary Therapies in Geriatric Practice: Selected Topics* (ed: Ann Burkhardt, and Jodi Carlson) The Haworth Press, Inc., 2001, pp. 23-34. Single or multiple copies of this article are available for a fee from The Haworth Document Delivery Service [1-800-342-9678, 9:00 a.m. - 5:00 p.m. (EST). E-mail address: getinfo@ haworthpressinc.com].

23

of the application and training principles involved with this age group, and research findings on the efficacy of this intervention.

Alternative therapies are becoming increasingly popular in clinical practice and recreational pursuits. One of the better known is the practice of Tai Chi Chuan. The primary goal of Tai Chi is to provide an avenue for the development of the body's natural rhythm and coordination and to harmonize those actions with deep relaxed breathing, mental focus, and specific patterns of movement (O'Connor & Lane, 1999).

HISTORY

In order to fully encompass an understanding of Tai Chi and how it has come to be so widely used for health, recreation, and self-defense purposes, some reference to its history and origins would be helpful. There are many alternative spellings of this martial art form, and it may be referred to as Taiji, Taijiquan, T'ai Chi, T'ai Chi Chuan, or Tai Chi Chuan. In literal translation, T'ai Chi means "the grand ultimate first" (Cerrato, 1999) and Chuan means "fist" (Wolf et al., 1997).

Tai Chi has a rich and long heritage spanning more than four thousand years. There are several different historical references and some debate as to the true origins of the practice of Tai Chi. The first apparent written reference to T'ai Chi appeared in the *Book of Changes*, or the *I Ching* (Wilhelm & Baynes, 1967), approximately 3000 years ago with the following quotation from Cheng and Smith (1987): "Nature is always in motion. Man also should strengthen himself without interruption" (p. 1). Approximately 700 years ago, Chang San-feng, a Chinese martial artist and legendary Taoist priest of the Yuan dynasty (1279-1368), is credited with having developed Tai Chi as a form of self defense for monks (Cheng & Smith, 1987; Cheng, 1999). He reputedly obtained his inspiration from observing a fight between a crane and a snake (Koh, 1981) or through a dream (Cheng & Smith, 1987). Another source attributes the origin of Tai Chi to the T'ang Dynasty between the years 618 and 907 (Cheng & Smith, 1987).

According to Liao (1990), the search for a constructive and harmonious way to realize the full potential of the human spirit and the body's natural balance began a few hundred years ago with the development of the Tai Chi exercise system. However, there is no clearly defined historical reference for the beginning of this balanced body and mind system. The present practice may be only 300 years old (Wolf et al., 1997). Tai Chi Chuan was also known as "shadow boxing" (Koh, 1981; O'Connor &

Lane, 1999) and was developed from a defensive martial art for protection from invaders (Chinese Sports Editorial Board, 1986). It is a traditional Chinese conditioning exercise form and has been practiced in the Orient for centuries as a form of relaxation, dance, and as a religious and spiritual ritual. It combines a program of mind-body exercises with mental and physical benefits to the practitioners. Tai Chi embodies the theory of the complementarity of the opposite qualities of yin (dark, cold, yielding, passivity, constructive, feminine) and yang (light, heat, action, destructive, masculine). Tai Chi is based on the Taoist belief that balanced energy, chi or life force, results in good health.

Traditionally, instruction in Tai Chi started out as a master-to-student apprenticeship, usually strictly within the same family. The information was passed down through the generations by observation, emulation, and by word of mouth rather than by any form of written record. The lessons often took place in the home of the respective masters from whose lineage various forms of Tai Chi evolved. The Chen style originated from that family who lived in a small village in Hopeh Province and is supposedly the precursor of all the other styles of Tai Chi. The Yang style evolved from the Chen style by the teaching that Yang Lu-ch'an received from the grandmaster of the Chen family. This was an unusual break from the traditional family lineage instruction, and Yang brought this practice to Beijing (Chia & Goh, 1986). Other styles (such as Sun, Hao, and Wu) developed, or were adapted, from the Yang style.

Originally there were 13 basic movements or postures in Tai Chi. Using these basic movements, the various styles have added somewhere between 14 and 119 more postures to those original numbers. The contemporary Yang style long form of Tai Chi has 108 separate and distinct moves, some of which are frequently repeated throughout the entire sequence. However, the ideal practice is to combine all the moves imperceptibly in a graceful series of flowing bodily movements which are integrated by focused mental concentration, slow breathing, the gradual shifting of the weight from side to side and forwards and backwards, and by relaxation of the muscles not involved. Several style variations of this traditional long form of 108 moves have evolved over the intervening years. For example, it was shortened to 37 postures by Cheng Man-ch'ing with the blessing of his master teacher, Yang Cheng-fu. Cheng Man-ch'ing brought these 37 postures to the USA, omitting a lot of the repetitive movements that are common in the longer form. He also developed the abbreviated eight methods which cover the basics of Tai Chi, to help older people and those with limited practice time to gain the benefits of Tai Chi Chuan (Cheng & Smith, 1987).

These adapted short forms have made Tai Chi more manageable and appealing to the general public because of the gentle, repetitive, and flowing movements of the body which are accompanied by deep diaphragmatic breathing (Cerrato, 1999). This concentrated attention and general awareness of rhythm and form leads the practitioner into a state of peaceful mindfulness.

The Western world considered Tai Chi and other modified martial art forms to be strange behaviors 30 years ago. However, they are now considered to be part of a readily accepted form of physical exercise and mental discipline and are gaining popularity and media visibility. Tai Chi is deeply rooted in the traditional Chinese culture, and many elderly Chinese people perform Tai Chi as part of a personal daily centering ritual in their parks, lakesides, and mountains each morning in a quiet, dedicated manner. In certain areas of the United States where there is a large Chinese population, this practice has been observed taking place in school playgrounds, parks, beaches, and other open spaces.

Tai Chi is a low impact, non-competitive exercise which incorporates a contemplative inner focus, possibly enhancing and maintaining optimal health, potentially increasing longevity, and also providing techniques for self-defense (Koh, 1981). It promotes correct postural alignment, mental clarity, and deep and relaxed breathing. Other additional benefits include greater flexibility, improved muscular strength, coordination, muscle control, promoting relaxation, and reducing mental stress (Berg, 1995; Birkel, 1998; Daley & Spinks, 2000; Wolf, Barnhart, Ellison, & the Atlanta FICSIT Group, 1997). It is a series of gradual movements that follow flowing, rotational, forward, and sideways reaching movements of the trunk and limbs. It is comprised of a series of precise, structured body positions, likened to those of animals and birds, which flow together as a continuous sequence of unbroken movements when practiced in the completed form (Baer, 1997).

Many of the Tai Chi forms are based on the laws of nature; for example, the lower body is firmly rooted on the ground and the upper body moves gently like clouds in the wind. Several of the postures relate to animals in the translation from the Chinese, such as "Repulse Monkey," "White Crane Spreads Wings," and "Parting the Wild Horse's Mane" (Argo, 1998). These movements appear effortless to the casual observer but in fact require considerable mental concentration and physical coordination (Baer, 1997; Yan, 1995; Yan, 1998).

The slow and controlled movements of Tai Chi minimize undue stress on the joints and connective tissues of the body which are important considerations for the older adult. These slow and gentle movements of Tai Chi are similar in many respects to proprioceptive neuromuscular facilitation techniques as they involve large muscular movement patterns in diagonal and rotational patterns around the horizontal axis of the spine (Basmajian, 1984; Levandoski & Leyshon, 1990).

Our modern Western society typically rewards and emphasizes speed of task accomplishment and the attainment of some form of instant gratification. Tai Chi provides the opposite rewards of quiet contemplation, of freedom from the stresses of everyday life, from chronic pain and illness, fatigue, anxiety, depression, confusion, and physical instability (Jin, 1989, 1992). If Tai Chi principles of thoughtful, focused movements were emulated in rising from sitting and moving slowly with focused attention, there may be fewer incidents of physical trauma from balance loss and falls.

TAI CHI APPLICATION TO THE PROBLEMS OF ELDERLY PEOPLE

Many problems with which elderly people have to contend are ideally addressed in Tai Chi practice. Some of these typical problems include decreased mobility, general weakness, osteoporosis, poor coordination and balance, decline in maximal oxygen uptake, slowed mental and physical reaction time to external stimuli, social isolation, depression, and fatigue (O'Connor & Lane, 1999; Daley & Spinks, 2000).

There could be significant advantages to our national economy in implementing rehabilitation and prevention programs to reduce some of these age-related factors. Falls among elderly people are one of the most common health risks and can be attributed to environmental, biomechanical, physiological, and psychological events (Kessenich, 1998; Tinetti, Speechley, & Ginter, 1988). One researcher (Jin, 1989) found that Tai Chi practice may have psychological benefits in reducing the levels of tension, anxiety, depression, anger, confusion, mood disturbance, and fatigue.

According to Tinetti et al. (1988), 30% of community dwelling adults over the age of 65 have at least one fall per year. This incidence increases to 40% in those over the age of 80 years. The most common precursors to falls in elderly people occur in dynamic situations of routine activities of daily living, such as standing, walking, descending stairs, and picking up objects from the floor (Alexander, 1994). Predictable consequences of falls in this age group include fractures, hospitalizations, and death as a result of the numerous complications of inactivity, immobility, and infection. For these reasons, interventions are needed that will potentially reduce the significant incidence of falls in this age group. The scientific research conducted on some of these aspects will be discussed later in this article.

TAI CHI TRAINING

Tai Chi is a non-competitive activity and can be practiced by people of any age after simple instructions have been given. It is essential for prospective students to study the various Tai Chi forms with a knowledgeable and patient instructor, especially as these intricate movements are generally unfamiliar to most westerners. Typical classes involve repeated and specific verbal instructions and physical demonstrations that provide a framework for the student's proficiency in executing the movements. Participants concentrate on the performance of the slow, graceful, sequential Tai Chi movements, producing mental and physical relaxation which help to reduce external distractions (Yan, 1995). However, most elderly students have to overcome the frustration of easy distractibility, of being unable to remember the sequence of the moves, having a poor sense of balance, and the overall weakness of the lower body muscles.

The Tai Chi practitioner begins by focusing on slow, calm breathing. The feet are separated with the spine held erect, the knees are bent slightly, and there is a settling of the torso into the hip joints. The deeper the legs are bent, the more challenging the postures become due to an increased demand on the sustaining muscles of the thighs (Wolfson et al., 1996). The arms are gracefully raised in front and lowered in unison with the breath, and the weight is then shifted from one foot to the other, following a predetermined series of movements. The movements of the upper extremities tend to be slow, circular, and flowing from the waist. The trunk movements encourage erect posture and increased rotation while the movements of the lower extremities focus on stability, strength, and balance. These aspects are attained in moves that involve a lower "sitting" posture in which there is a greater degree of knee and hip flexion (Wolfson et al., 1996).

The regular practice of low-impact, modified Tai Chi exercise may be accomplished in as little as 10 minutes a day. Sedentary elderly people often have a decline in cardiorespiratory function and fail to use the full excursion of the lungs' capacity for optimal metabolism of oxygen (Lan, Lai, Wong, & Yu, 1996). For this reason the inclusion of slow and deep breathing is particularly beneficial. In the exhalation phase of the breath (yang), the upper body movements are in the forward and upward direction and in the inhalation phase (yin), they are downwards and back (Kessenich, 1998). This form of safe, aerobic exercise has been found appropriate for the older age group (Tsai & Chen, 1996). Some additional self-reported benefits attributed to Tai Chi practice include restoration of optimal health and tranquillity, tension relief, energy regeneration, increased flexibility and strength, inner calmness, stress reduction, mental acuity, and improved balance (Kutner, Barnhart, Wolf, McNeely, & Xu, 1997; Tse & Bailey, 1992; Wolf et al., 1996).

Improving balance, strength, and flexibility are most applicable to the goals of rehabilitation of impaired and well-functioning elderly people by physical and occupational therapists. It is important to find a way to motivate elderly people in order to insure their ongoing use of an appropriate and beneficial exercise program. It has been this author's clinical observation that many elderly people tend to think of exercise as arduous, painful, or unpleasant. Other authors cite psychosocial factors influencing and limiting exercise participation in this age group for reasons of perceived age-inappropriate behavior (Ostrow, Jones, & Spiker, 1981; Ostrow & Dzewaltowski, 1986). Tai Chi may provide the benefits of social interaction, a sense of enjoyment and accomplishment, as well as a sense of subjectively "feeling better," and, therefore, it may become a pleasurable, ongoing activity (Wolf et al., 1997). Once mastered, Tai Chi can be practiced anywhere at any time independent of the need for fine weather, special clothing or equipment, or a special environment. Memorizing a detailed routine and then reproducing it through the movements of the body can increase the practitioner's sense of self-esteem (Birkel, 1998). Conversely, however, the frustrations of being unable to recall the specific moves temporarily may have the opposite effect.

In Tai Chi there are twisting and pivoting steps and stances that may require prolonged bending of the hips and knees. One of the movements requires marked concentration on coordinating walking backwards together with forward movements of the arms. These slow movements and the inner concentration involved can help to increase awareness of the instability that could precede a fall. An overall awareness of balance is attained by the lowered placement of the body's center of gravity located below the navel and between the abdomen and the spine. When the focus is on this area, and the moves are all initiated from the conscious awareness of this place, the individual is much more difficult to uproot, tip over, or be knocked off balance. Some of the moves or postures require a narrower stance that gradually reduces the base of support to a single limb stance (Wolf et al., 1996). Other postures demand a wider upper-body reach in forward or diagonal directions. These duplicate some of the daily functional positions in which there is a tendency to lose balance (Duncan, Weiner, Chandler, & Studenski, 1990).

EVIDENCE OF EFFICACY

The Chinese government was apparently aware of the health benefits associated with the regular practice of Tai Chi and initiated a standardized maintenance program in 1949 (Rappaport, 1999). However, it was not until the 1980s that Chinese scientists began to investigate the potential and actual benefits of Tai Chi (Forge, 1997). That year also provided the first documented study in the Western scientific literature of the physiological responses accompanying the practice of Tai Chi (Brown, Mucci, Hetzler, & Knowlton, 1989). Subsequent research studies have pointed towards the increased benefit that can be attained by complementing more orthodox therapeutic interventions with the inclusion of Tai Chi practice. For example, 38 senior adults were included in an 8-week study involving the practice of Tai Chi with the control group participants walking or jogging. It was found that the Tai Chi group demonstrated better motor control, balance, and greater fluidity of arm movements (Downing & Yan, 1998). The researchers attributed these findings of improved balance to the ability of the participants in the Tai Chi group to utilize sensory feedback by the slow and deliberate training process, the focus on the movement sensations, and the relaxation and breathing that accompanies the practice of the forms.

Lumsden, Baccala, and Martire (1998) have investigated the use of Tai Chi for patients with osteoarthritis. They reported that these patients had improved balance and muscle strength and did not find this form of exercise to increase the deterioration of the bone or to be any more stressful on the weight bearing joints than other forms of prescribed exercise which incorporate standing movements or impact on the body. Patients with rheumatoid arthritis also found that 10 weeks of Tai Chi practice did not exacerbate joint damage or swelling (Kirsteins, Dietz, & Hwang, 1991), unlike some other forms of exercise.

Several researchers have investigated the factors of balance, flexibility, and lower extremity strength as they relate to the prevention of falls and the serious consequences (Gehlsen & Whaley, 1990; Tse & Bailey, 1992; Forsythe, 1996; Wolfson et al., 1996; Wolf et al., 1996). It has been estimated that the consequences of falls leading to fractures, hospitalizations, and death from the numerous complications of inactivity, immobility, and infection in the elderly cost the economy in excess of $10 billion per year. Over 300,000 people per year experience hip fractures that may be due in part to impaired balance as well as to other medical factors, such as osteoporosis (Wolf et al., 1996). O'Connor and Lane (1999) report Tai Chi practitioners in the elderly age group have 47% fewer falls and a 75% reduction in the incidence of hip fractures in comparison to a group who did not participate in Tai Chi.

Lan and colleagues (1996) studied the aspect of cardiorespiratory function in a group of independent community dwellers. Some of these people had been practicing Tai Chi for approximately 5 years, and some were sedentary with no participation in any form of physical exercise for the same 5-year period. These researchers found a significant increase in the peak exercise oxygen uptake in both men and women in the Tai Chi group when compared to the sedentary group. Additionally, the Tai Chi group demonstrated greater physical flexibility and a lower percentage of body fat when compared to the sedentary group. In a later study Lan et al. (1999) evaluated the training effect of a one-year program of Tai Chi on a group of low-risk patients who had previously undergone coronary artery bypass surgery. The results indicated that this type of intervention increased the maximal aerobic capacity of the Tai Chi group by approximately 10% over the non-directed exercise group.

In 1990, the National Institute on Aging began sponsoring research in a special frailty reduction program. Specific research projects involving the use of T'ai Chi with the elderly population were published in May of 1996. The first was conducted by Steven L. Wolf, PhD, senior Taiji instructor Dr. Tingsen Xu, and their colleagues at Emory University School of Medicine in Atlanta, Georgia. They instructed 200 elderly people, with an average age of approximately 76 years, in a 15-week program. The subjects were divided into three groups that received one of the following: instruction in Tai Chi, computerized balance training, or balance education. They found a statistically significant difference in the group practicing Tai Chi in which there was a 47.5% reduction in the risk of multiple falls while the other two group interventions proved to be less effective.

The second study by Leslie Wolfson, MD, and his colleagues (1996) at the University of Connecticut Health Center in Farmington used a combination of several interventions to improve balance and strength in the elderly population. Outcome data from that study indicated that the experimental group subjects who continued to practice Tai Chi on a regular basis maintained the improvement in strength and balance after the 6-month follow-up period.

Huffman (1999) reviewed a study by Young, Appel, Jee, and Miller (1999) in which the effects of Tai Chi and modified aerobic exercise on decreasing blood pressure in a group of 60 to 80 year old people were investigated. The average exercise heart rate in the Tai Chi group was lower (75 beats per minute) than the aerobic group (112 beats per minute). It was concluded that low intensity activity might have antihypertensive effects on the sedentary elderly.

If the ability to reduce the number of falls was achieved by the regular use of a simple and inexpensive discipline, pain and suffering could be alleviated, and perhaps lives and health care dollars could be saved. Further research is needed for a thorough evaluation of the use of Tai Chi in health-related fields. The studies that have been published so far have indicated some of the benefits attained by this practice, but they have been of short duration and the sample sizes generally have been small (Chen & Snyder, 1999). It would seem to be desirable for our aging population to find effective methods to remain physically active and to have an increased quality of life as measured by the ability to continue to be safely independent, and to be generally less stressed.

In summary, Tai Chi is an appropriate form of exercise for an elderly population that frequently remains sedentary. Balance and coordination are improved, cardiovascular function is enhanced, stress is reduced, and falls may be prevented (Lan et al., 1996; Yan, 1995; O'Connor & Lane, 1999). Incorporating Tai Chi practice in an enjoyable, brief, daily routine is one way to attain an independent life and the health benefits accompanying this ancient oriental practice.

REFERENCES

Alexander, N. (1994). Postural control in older adults. *Journal of the American Geriatrics Society, 42,* 93-108.

Argo, C. (1998). Water Tai Chi. *American Fitness, 16*(4), 52-53.

Baer, K. (1997). A movement towards t'ai chi. *Harvard Health Letter, 22*(9), 6.

Basmajian, J. (Ed.) (1984). *Therapeutic exercise.* Baltimore: Williams and Wilkins.

Berg, R. (1995). Cerebral fitness. *Working Woman, 20*(2), 60.

Birkel, D. (1998). Activities for the older adult: Integration of the body and the mind. *Journal of Physical Education, Recreation and Dance, 69*(9), 23-28.

Brown, D., Mucci, W., Hetzler, R., & Knowlton, R. (1989). Cardiovascular and ventilatory responses during formalized Tai Chi Chuan exercise. *Research Quarterly for Exercise and Sport, 60*(3), 246-250.

Cerrato, P. (1999). Tai chi: A martial art turns therapeutic. *RN, 62*(2), 59.

Chen, K., & Snyder, M. (1999). A research-based use of Tai Chi/movement therapy as a nursing intervention. *Journal of Holistic Nursing, 17*(3), 267-279.

Cheng, J. (1999). Tai Chi Chuan: A slow dance for health. *The Physician and Sports Medicine, 27*(6), 9.

Cheng, M., & Smith, R. (1987). *T`ai-Chi: The "supreme ultimate" exercise for health, sport, and self-defense.* Vermont: Tuttle.

Chia, S., & Goh, E. (1986). *Tai Chi; ten minutes to health.* Sebastopol, CA: CRCS Publications.

Chinese Sports Editorial Board. (1986). *Simplified Taijiquan.* Bejing, China: Foreign Languages Printing House.

Daley, M., & Spinks, W. (2000). Exercise, mobility and aging. *Sports Medicine, 1,* 1-12.

Downing, J., & Yan, J. (1998). The effects of Tai Chi and traditional locomotor exercises on senior citizens' motor control. *Journal of Physical Education, Recreation and Dance, 69*(9), 9.

Duncan, P., Weiner, D., Chandler, J., & Studenski, S. (1999). Functional reach: A new measure of clinical balance. *Journal of Gerontology, 45,* 192-197.

Forge, R. (1997). Mind-body fitness: Encouraging prospects for primary and secondary prevention. *Journal of Cardiovascular Nursing, 11*(3), 53-65.

Forsythe, T. (1996). Using T`ai Chi to prevent falls in senior citizens. *Journal of Traditional Eastern Health and Fitness, 6*(1), 30-35.

Gehlsen, G., & Whaley, M. (1990). Falls in the elderly: Part I, gait; S in the elderly: Part II, balance, strength, and flexibility. *Archives of Physical Medicine and Rehabilitation, 71,* 735-741.

Huffman, G. (1999). Aerobic activity versus T`ai Chi: Effects on blood pressure. *American Family Physician, 60*(3), 980.

Jin, P. (1989). Changes in heart rate, noradrenaline, cortisol and mood during Tai Chi. *Journal of Psychosomatic Research, 33*(2), 197-206.

Jin, P. (1992). Efficacy of Tai Chi, brisk walking, meditation, and reading in reducing mental and emotional stress. *Journal of Psychosomatic Research, 36*(4), 361-70.

Kessenich, C. (1998). Tai Chi as a method of fall prevention in the elderly. *Orthopedic Nursing, 17*(4), 27.

Kirsteins, A., Dietz, F., & Hwang, S. (1991). Evaluating the safety and potential use of a weight bearing exercise, tai chi chuan, for rheumatoid arthritis patients. *American Journal of Physical Medicine and Rehabilitation, 70*(3), 136.

Koh, T. (1981). Tai Chi Chuan. *American Journal of Chinese Medicine, 9,* 15-22.

Kutner, N., Barnhart, H., Wolf, S., McNeely, E., & Xu, T. (1997). Self-report benefits of Tai Chi practice by older adults. *Journal of Gerontology, 52*(5), 242-246.

Lan, C., Chen, S., Lai, J., & Wong, M. (1999). The effect of Tai Chi on cardiorespiratory function in patients with coronary artery bypass surgery. *Medicine Science Sports Exercise, 31*(5), 634-638.

Lan, C., Lai, J., Wong, M., & Yu, M. (1996). Cardiorespiratory function, flexibility, and body composition among geriatric Tai Chi Chuan practitioners. *Archive of Physical Medicine and Rehabilitation, 77*(6), 612-616.

Levandoski, L., & Leyshon, G. (1990). Tai Chi exercise and the elderly. *Clinical Kinesiology, 44* (2), 39-42.

Liao, W. (1990). *T'ai Chi classics.* Boston: Shambala.

Lumsden, D., Baccala, A., & Martire, J. (1998). Tai Chi for osteoarthritis: An introduction for primary care physicians. *Geriatrics, 53*(2), 84.

O'Connor, W., & Lane, J. (1999). Benefits of Tai Chi in Osteoporosis. *American Journal of Medicine & Sports, 1*(5), 255-259.

Ostrow, A., & Dzewaltowski, D. (1986). Older adults perceptions of physical activity participation based on age-role and sex-role appropriateness. *Research Quarterly for Exercise and Sport, 57,* 167-169.

Ostrow, A., Jones, D., & Spiker, D. (1981). Age role expectations and sex role expectations for selected sports activities. *Research Quarterly for Exercise and Sport, 52,* 216-217.

Rappaport, J. (1999). Muscle and meditation: The ancient art of Tai Chi builds strength–and serenity–in a few minutes a day. *Natural Health, 27*(2), 106.

Tinetti, M., Speechley, M., & Ginter, S. (1988). Risk factors for falls among elderly persons living in the community. *New England Journal of Medicine, 319,* 1701-1707.

Tsai, C., & Chen, J. (1996). Physiological responses to Tai Chi Chuan exercise in middle-aged and elderly males. *Taoyuan, Taiwan: Graduate Institute of Sports Science, National College of Physical Education and Sports.*

Tse, S., & Bailey, D. (1992). Tai Chi and postural control in the well elderly. *American Journal of Occupational Therapy, 46,* 295-300.

Wilhelm, R., & Baynes, C. (1967). *The I Ching or Book of Changes.* Bollingen Series XIX. Princeton: Princeton University Press.

Wolf, S., Barnhart, H., Ellison, G., & the Atlanta FICSIT Group. (1997). The effects of Tai Chi Quan and computerized balance training on postural stability in older subjects. *Physical Therapy, 4,* 385-394.

Wolf, S., Barnhart, H., Kutner, N., McNeely, E., Coogler, C., & Xu, T. (1996). Reducing frailty and falls in older persons: An investigation of Tai Chi and computerized balance training. *Journal of the American Geriatrics Society, 44*(5), 489-497.

Wolf, S., Coogler, C., & Xu, T. (1997). Exploring the basis for Tai Chi Chuan as a therapeutic exercise approach. *Archives of Physical Medicine and Rehabilitation, 78,* 886-892.

Wolfson, L., Wipple, R., Derby, C., Judge, J., King, M., Amerman, P., Schmidt, J., & Smyers, D. (1996). Balance and strength training in older adults: Intervention gains and Tai Chi maintenance. *Journal of the American Geriatrics Society, 44*(5), 498-506.

Yan, J. (1995). The health and fitness benefits of tai chi. *The Journal of Physical Education and Dance, 66*(9), 61.

Yan, J. (1998). Tai Chi practice improves senior citizens' balance and arm movement control. *Journal of Aging and Physical Activity, 6,* 271-284.

Young, D., Appel, L., Jee, S., & Miller, E. III. (1999). The effects of aerobic exercise and T'ai Chi on blood pressure in older people: Results of a randomized trial. *Journal of the American Geriatrics Society, 47*(3), 277-284.

Energy Therapies
for Physical and Occupational Therapists
Working with Older Adults

Ellen Zambo Anderson, PT, MA, GCS

SUMMARY. The National Center for Complementary and Alternative Medicine (NCCAM) has begun to identify, define, and categorize complementary and alternative healing practices. The purpose of this article is to explore approaches of health and healing that are based on the assumption that subtle energy fields exist within and around the human body. Basic theories, rationales, and evidence for Qigong, Polarity Therapy, Reiki, and Therapeutic Touch will be reviewed. Applications and implications for the physical and occupational therapist working with older adults will also be discussed. *[Article copies available for a fee from The Haworth Document Delivery Service: 1-800-342-9678. E-mail address: <getinfo@haworthpressinc.com> Website: <http://www.HaworthPress.com> © 2001 by The Haworth Press, Inc. All rights reserved.]*

KEYWORDS. Energy therapy, Qigong, polarity therapy, Reiki, therapeutic touch, occupational therapy, physical therapy

As people get older, they begin to realize that the aging process affects more than one's physiological state. Frequently, aging is accom-

Ellen Zambo Anderson is Assistant Professor of Physical Therapy at the University of Medicine and Dentistry of New Jersey–School of Allied Health Professions, 65 Bergen Street, Newark, NJ 07107-3301.

[Haworth co-indexing entry note]: "Energy Therapies for Physical and Occupational Therapists Working with Older Adults." Anderson, Ellen Zambo. Co-published simultaneously in *Physical & Occupational Therapy in Geriatrics* (The Haworth Press, Inc.) Vol. 18, Number 4, 2001, pp. 35-49; and: *Complementary Therapies in Geriatric Practice: Selected Topics* (ed: Ann Burkhardt, and Jodi Carlson) The Haworth Press, Inc., 2001, pp. 35-49. Single or multiple copies of this article are available for a fee from The Haworth Document Delivery Service [1-800-342-9678, 9:00 a.m. - 5:00 p.m. (EST). E-mail address: getinfo@haworthpressinc.com].

panied by a shift in one's socioeconomic status in which changes in finances, living environment, and social/family supports may be new concerns (Guccione, 1993). In addition, elders face health issues such as physical illness, chronic pain, and disability to a greater extent than the younger population. The combination of these social and physical conditions give rise to the notion that nearly all problems faced by the elderly will have a physiological and psychological component (Dossey, 1997). Perhaps in an effort to address the multidimensional issues of rehabilitation and health in the elderly, health care professionals have begun to investigate interventions that propose to address both body and mind (Sancier, 1996; Scott, 1999; Wolf, Barnhart, Ellison, and Coogler, 1997). Another consideration may be that health care professionals are beginning to follow the consumer's lead. According to Eisenberg, Kessler, Foster, Norlock, Calkins, and Delbanco (1993), in 1990, one-third of adult Americans consulted non-conventional health care providers and spent more than fourteen billion dollars for that care. Over ten billion dollars of that money was spent out of pocket.

Of particular interest to many therapists (McCormack & Galantino, 1997; Selby, 1997; Sharp, 1997) is the area of mind-body medicine that considers the use of subtle energy flow as a mechanism for facilitating optimum function, health, and well being. This article will explore the theories, rationales, evidence, and application of some approaches that acknowledge subtle energy fields of the body and promote manipulation of such fields for optimal health. Implications for physical and occupational therapists working with geriatric patients will also be discussed.

To address the question of how mind-body or energy therapies differ from "traditional" physical and occupational therapies, one needs to explore the difference between Western medicine and Chinese or Eastern medicine. Becker and Selden (1985) and Gerber (1988) have explained the foundation of Western medicine as being "mechanistic" in nature. Human physiological and psychological behavior is viewed to be dependent on the structure of the brain and body. The heart, for example, is a mechanical pump and the kidneys are an automatic filtration system. Much emphasis in health care has, therefore, been placed on surgical techniques to remove, replace, or repair body parts that are not working properly. Drug therapy, although somewhat different in philosophy, is also based on this mechanistic view. Instead of scalpels, physicians use pharmacological interventions to strengthen or destroy cells not functioning appropriately.

Other systems of medicine, such as traditional Chinese medicine and Ayurvedic medicine, see human beings as multidimensional organisms made up of dynamic, interactive energy systems. This energetic network, which represents the physical/cellular framework, is nurtured by a vital energy known as "qi" or "ch'i" in Chinese, "prana" in Sanskrit, and "ki" in Japanese. Body and mind are viewed as being inextricably connected via these energy systems, and it is considered that a healthy state is achieved when all systems are in balance and the energy of life can flow freely. Another concept important to Eastern medicine is that of universal polarity. Traditional Chinese medicine assumes that energy moves and is transformed by virtue of the tension between electromagnetic fields with opposite poles. The negative pole, known as the yin, and the positive pole, known as the yang, is acknowledged in all forms of energy including matter. According to the *Yellow Emperor's Classic of Internal Medicine*, a medical treatise written at least 2,000 years ago, and still an indispensable text of Chinese medicine, "the entire universe is an oscillation of the forces of yin and yang" (Veith, 1970).

In keeping with traditional Chinese medicine, a healthy organism is one that has adequate Qi with an even balance of the yin and yang energy forces. An imbalance of energies causes a shift in the equilibrium of the organism that can create patterns of disharmony and illness (Reid, 1994). Qi energy is absorbed from the universe through the skin via portals that are said to have reduced electrical resistance (Gordon, 1997; Gerber, 1988). These areas are now commonly known as acupuncture points and are found along a specialized meridian system that runs deep below the integument to the underlying organ structures (Gerber, 1988; Reid, 1994). It is by twelve pairs of major organ meridians that Qi flows into the organs to provide life-sustaining energy. Although the mechanism by which acupuncture appears to be helpful in promoting health and well being is not completely understood, its acceptance into Western medical practice has grown widely since the 1970s (Helms, 1998).

Despite the growing acceptance of acupuncture in the Western world, other interventions that acknowledge a mind-body connection or subtle energy flow have not met with such acceptance. Perhaps this is partially due to the limited number of experimental studies conducted in the West with the purpose of investigating the mechanism and efficacy of such therapies (Dossey, 1995).

With the recent inception of the National Center for Complementary and Alternative Medicine (NCCM), however, greater attention is now being focused on defining the issues of complementary approaches in health care and establishing a research agenda. NCCAM (2000) defined mind-body medicine as involving "behavioral, psychological, social and spiritual approaches to health," such as Yoga, Qigong, and Tai Chi. "Behavioral medicine," as defined by NCCAM, refers to practices that fall mainly within the domains of conventional medicine, such as psychotherapy, meditation, imagery, hypnosis, biofeedback and support groups. Overlapping practices are those that can be either complementary of alternative medicine (CAM) or behavioral medicine, depending on its application. These approaches include art therapy, music therapy, dance therapy, journaling, humor, and body psychotherapy (NCCAM, 2000).

Additional interventions with assumptions of subtle energy flow and balance are listed within the NCCAM classification system as either "Manipulative and Body-Base Systems" or "Biofield." "Manipulative and Body-Based Systems" are defined as "systems that are based on manipulation and/or movement of the body" and include Polarity Therapy, an approach based on the concept of releasing blocked life energy via manual manipulation (Sharp, 1997). Other approaches within this category are: Trager, Alexander, Feldenkrais, Pilates and Rolfing. "Biofield" is defined by NCCAM (2000) as medicine that involves ". . . systems that use subtle energy fields in and around the body for medical purposes." Some approaches listed are Therapeutic Touch, Reiki, and SHEN (NCCAM, 2000). This article will review the theories, research, and the possible application of some energy-based approaches that are gaining interest and popularity in Western culture and medicine.

QIGONG

As previously stated, "Qi" is Chinese for "life" or "vital energy." "Gong" refers to work, skill, or training. It, therefore, follows that Qigong is an approach that promotes one's ability to control his or her energy thereby ensuring a harmonious balance of energy and wellness (Reid, 1994). Although there are many approaches to Qigong, the basis for every approach is the combination of deep, diaphragmatic breathing with slow, flowing movements (Dong & Esser, 1990). Reid (1994) suggests that the psychophysiological effect of these combined activities "is to switch the autonomic nervous system from the chronically overactive sympathetic mode to the calming, restorative parasympathetic mode" (p. 180).

In China, Qigong has long been considered by many to be a way of life that has many anti-aging benefits (Ankun, Chongxing, Dinghi, &

Yuesheng, 1991). Unfortunately, much of the research on Qigong has been performed in China, making it difficult to translate and interpret (Luskin, Newell, Griffith, Holmes, Telles, Manasti, Pelletier, & Haskell, 1998). Wu, Bandilla, Ciccone, Yang, Cheng, Carner, Wu, and Shen (1999) have identified three areas of Qigong investigation, all written or presented in Chinese. These areas include: (1) effects of Qi emission on chemical and physical properties of various substances and sensors; (2) effects of Qi emission on living cells; and (3) human studies involving Qigong training.

Kenneth Sancier of the Qigong Institute in San Francisco has summarized much of this research, focusing on the healthful benefits of Qigong in addressing hypertension, dementia, and stress (Sancier, 1996a, 1996b). In one 20-year controlled study reviewed by Sancier (1996a), the researchers concluded that Qigong was an effective intervention for hypertension as evidenced by a reduction of dosage of an antihypertensive drug and a 50% decrease in both mortality and morbidity from strokes. Another study Sancier (1996a) reviewed compared the effects of Qigong with walking or running and found that the subjects who practiced Qigong for 6 months had a reduction in 8 of the 14 clinical signs used to describe dementia. In a study by Ryu, Jun, Lee, Choi, Kim, and Chung (1995) Qigong was shown to have a positive effect on stress reduction with a possible link to immune function as evidenced by an increase in the number of T-lymphocyte cells measured in persons participating in Qigong.

Qigong's combination of non-impact, slow movements, and deep breathing appears to be a low risk intervention for promoting health and well being. Preliminary findings support Qigong as being beneficial for chronic conditions found in the elderly, including hypertension, coronary artery disease, and arthritis (Luskin et al., 1998). Further research is required, however, to answer many questions regarding this approach, including those that focus on Qigong's assumptions. Lines of inquiry to assess whether good health is dependent on an adequate and balanced energy flow and whether energy flow can in fact be modulated are certainly warranted.

POLARITY THERAPY

Polarity Therapy was developed in the mid-1900s by Dr. Randolf Stone, a chiropractor, osteopathic physician, and naturopath. Through his study of traditional Chinese medicine, Ayurvedic healing, herbal remedies, and spiritualism, Stone developed an energetic healing approach that acknowledges the Chinese concepts of yin and yang, but is more directly derived from the concepts of Ayurveda medicine or that of ancient Hindu healing practices (Kitts, 1988). Vital energy or Qi is known as "prana" in the Hindu tradition and is thought to be part of an energy system that focuses on the body's energy centers known as "chakras" (Karagulla & Kunz, 1989). These chakras, meaning "wheels" in Sanskrit, are said to resemble whirling vortices of subtle energy and are located at seven points along a vertical line ascending from the base of the spine to the head (Kunz, 1991). Each chakra is associated with a particular nerve plexus and endocrine gland and is thought to function as a type of energy transformer (Gerber, 1998).

Stone proposed a dynamic relationship between positive and negative charges at every level of organization within the universe and suggested that the pulsation of energy between two oppositely charged poles is the basis for a life force or energy (Sills, 1990). Disease or illness is thought to be due to a disruption of energy flow, and so Polarity Therapy proposes to release blocked energy and manipulate energy flow between negative and positive charges (Sharp, 1997).

During a typical Polarity Therapy session, therapists will apply pressure, rock, and/or shake their clients to balance the recipient's energy flow (Kitts, 1988). Afterward, the therapist may advise the client on proper diet according to the Ayurveda tradition and recommend certain stretches or exercises that promote the balancing of energy (Claire, 1995). Proponents of Polarity Therapy report that this approach is beneficial in clients with pain, discomfort, and stress and that by balancing one's energy, the onset of an illness may be prevented (Sills, 1990). If an illness has already occurred, Polarity Therapy may accelerate healing (Claire, 1995). Unfortunately, despite the extensive body of writings left by Dr. Stone and the existence of the American Polarity Therapy Association, no experimental studies have been conducted on the efficacy of this healing approach. Benford, Talngagi, Burr Doss, Bossey, and Arnold (1999) have investigated the fluctuation of electromagnetic fields during Polarity Therapy treatment and found a reduction in gamma radiation at four different treatment sites, but the explanation and implications for such a reduction have not been elucidated. Despite the suggestion by a physical therapist that Polarity Therapy is an intervention easily incorporated into a physical therapy session (Sharp, 1997), the lack of evidence for this approach may warrant greater scrutiny by the physical and occupational therapists who frequently encounter patients with normal age-related changes in addition to multi-system disorders.

REIKI

Reiki is an ancient energetic healing practice that utilizes the lay-ing-on-of-hands (Horan, 1992). Literally, "Reiki" is the Japanese word for "universal life energy." Rediscovered by Dr. Mikao Usui, a Japanese monk educator, Reiki has its origins in ancient Tibetan Buddhist teachings (Claire, 1995). Similar to other healing approaches based on Asian systems of medicine, an underlying assumption of Reiki is that disharmony in one's subtle energy fields can result in physical or emotional dysfunction or illness (Horan, 1992). Intervention is therefore directed at affecting or modulating energy fields or flow.

What singles out Reiki from other forms of complementary healing practices is that a Reiki practitioner intends to channel vital energy from the universal energy field into the human energy field for the purpose of healing (Barnett & Chambers, 1996). In addition, Reiki does not require the practitioner to diagnose an energy imbalance or intend for a repatterning of the energy flow. Instead, "it is the client who is in charge, her cells drawing in the amount of energy needed to bring the mind/body back to homeostasis" (Barnett & Chambers, 1996, p. 22). The proponents of Reiki, therefore, believe that there are no contraindications for its use.

During a typical Reiki session, a practitioner will hold his/her hands gently on the client's body in ten to twenty different positions that cover the chakras, major organs, and glands. At each position, the practitioner acts as a channeler of universal energy to the receiver. Unlike other energy approaches, practitioners are required to go through a series of initiations, called "attunements," with a Reiki master. This attunement process is what empowers the Reiki practitioner to channel energy from the universe (Claire, 1995).

Reiki practitioners advocate the use of Reiki as an approach that complements conventional medical treatment based on anecdotal reports that highlight its effectiveness in controlling pain, lessening anxiety, promoting relaxation, and facilitating healing and recovery (Barnett & Chambers, 1996). There is, however, at the time of this writing a void of scientific support for Reiki due to the paucity of research in this area. Olson and Hanson (1997) published the results of a pilot study that assessed the usefulness of Reiki as an adjunct to pharmacological intervention for pain management. Although a significant reduction in pain was recorded following Reiki treatment at the time of this writing, the study was markedly limited by its lack of an inclusion criteria and control for dependent variables. Mansour, Beuche, Laing, Leis, and Nurse

(1999) acknowledged a paucity of controlled experimental studies of Reiki and suggested that research in the area should begin with placebo-controlled investigations. In their study, the researchers established a standardized procedure for real and placebo Reiki and recommended that this procedure be incorporated into randomized clinical trials to investigate the efficacy of Reiki (Mansour et al., 1999).

Reiki practitioners believe that it is just a matter of time before science is able to provide the evidence to support the practice of Reiki and, therefore, continue to strongly endorse its use as an adjuvant to traditional medicine (Barnett & Chambers, 1996). They point out that prayer is not being withheld even though there is limited scientific evidence to support this activity as a complementary approach for healing and recovery, and, therefore, Reiki should not be withheld (Barnett & Chambers, 1996).

Because there do not appear to be any contraindications for Reiki, and the patient is not asked to perform any physical activities during a Reiki session, many health care professionals have been incorporating Reiki into their practices (Barnett & Chambers, 1996; Horan, 1992). Physical and occupational therapists who use Reiki as a complement to traditional rehabilitation interventions such as strength and endurance training should be encouraged to develop a paradigm that includes a clinical decision making process by which one can determine the circumstances in which Reiki may be useful. Physical and occupational therapists should also consider identifying and incorporating assessment tools into their examinations that can be used to measure the proposed benefits of Reiki such as discomfort, anxiety, relaxation, and "healing." Then, we may be better able to identify the role Reiki does or does not play in achieving positive outcomes for the patient.

THERAPEUTIC TOUCH

Therapeutic Touch (TT) is a contemporary interpretation of several ancient health practices, one of which is the laying-on-of hands. Developed by Dolores Krieger, PhD, RN, professor emeritus at New York University and Dora Kunz, TT is a healing approach that is said to modulate or rebalance one's energy field (Krieger, 1979). Like other approaches previously discussed, TT practitioners believe that disease reflects an imbalance in the human energy field and that balancing one's energy field can support an individual's own power for self-healing. Unfortunately, the name "Therapeutic Touch" is somewhat misleading, because most often the practitioner holds his/her hands several inches away from the client to assess and modulate the client's energy field. Frequently, the practitioner never even "touches" the client. Krieger developed TT through her observations of healers throughout the world and her knowledge of Asian medical systems. Specifically, Krieger (1993) based many of the principles of TT on the ancient Hindu concepts of prana and chakras and proposes that every human being is an open energy system. This assumption implies that every person's energy field extends beyond the physical body and is in constant interface with other energy fields (Krieger, 1993). Krieger (1997) has further suggested that the theoretical foundation of TT may be supported by the relatively new science of quantum physics, which deals with the emission and absorption of energy by matter (Capra, 1975). These concepts allow for the TT practitioner to be a modulator of energy flow and fields (Krieger, 1997).

A TT session typically lasts between twenty and thirty minutes depending on the needs of the client. As described by Krieger (1979), the process of performing TT involves four steps: centering, assessing, unruffling, and transferring or modulating energy. Centering requires the practitioner to achieve a state of quiet or stillness so that he/she can focus intention toward the client without distraction. During the assessment stage, the practitioner assesses the client's energy field to determine areas of imbalance, congestion, low energy flow, or heat. Unruffling is the unscientific, yet descriptive term used to describe the process by which a practitioner clears a client's energy field so that the energy feels free and flowing. The final step in the TT process is the transferring or modulation of energy that is performed by the practitioner. As with Reiki, the practitioner taps into universal energy and directs it to areas of energy depletion previously identified in the client. The intention for all TT sessions is to restore balance in the client's energy field, thereby promoting an environment for self-healing (Krieger, 1997).

As an energy healing technique, TT has received the most attention in the literature. In addition to many descriptive articles and anecdotal reports, numerous scientific studies have been published since the early 1980s. Heidt (1981), Olsen and Sneed (1995), and Simington and Laing (1993) all found that subjects who received TT demonstrated a significant decrease in anxiety. Other studies (Gordon, Merenstein, D'Amico, & Hudgens, 1998; Keller & Bzdek, 1986; Turner, Clark, Gauthier, & Williams, 1998) have demonstrated that TT has been effective for pain reduction when compared to "sham" TT. On the other hand, Eckes Peck

(1997) concluded that although both TT and progressive muscle relaxation (PMR) were effective interventions to decrease pain, PMR was more effective than TT.

Adding to the body of literature in the area of TT, Easter (1997), Spence and Olsen (1997), and Winstead-Fry and Kijek (1999) have written integrative review articles on the state of research on TT. Although the authors conclude that there appears to be evidence in support of TT for the reduction of pain and anxiety, further investigation of this intervention is warranted. Research issues raised as problems include the need for an operational definition of therapeutic touch, inadequate descriptions of the study sample, small sample sizes, and an over reliance on the State-Trait Anxiety Inventory as an outcome measure (Winstead-Fry & Kijek, 1999). Suggestions for additional research included efficacy studies with more broadly conceived outcome measures and the inclusion of subjects with definable pathology.

Two of the studies previously mentioned may be of particular interest to physical and occupational therapists working with older individuals. Eckes Peck (1997) investigated the effect of TT on pain in elders with degenerative arthritis. The 82 subjects who completed the study met the inclusion criteria of 55-99 years of age, non-institutionalized, confirmed diagnosis of degenerative arthritis beyond the acute inflammatory period of at least 6 months, chronic pain longer than 6 months duration, able to read and speak English, and cognitively able to complete the measurement instruments. In the study by Gordon, Merenstein, D'Amico, and Hudgens (1998), 27 subjects, with a mean age of approximately 65 years of age and a diagnosis of osteoarthritis of at least one knee, were divided into a treatment group (TT), placebo group (mock TT), and control group (no intervention). In both studies, subjects who received TT experienced a significant reduction in the pain as measured by either a visual analogue scale, McGill Pain Questionnaire or the West Haven-Yale Multidimensional Pain Inventory.

Attempting to refute TT as a valid health care intervention, Rosa, Rosa, Sarner, and Barrett (1998) conducted a study in which TT practitioners were asked to detect whether the experimenter's hand was closer to the practitioner's left or right hand. To prevent the experimenter's hands from being seen, the TT practitioners were asked to place their hands through two cutouts of a tall, opaque screen. Of the 280 trials that were conducted, the practitioners were correct 123 times (44%). The authors concluded that because the TT practitioners were unable to reliably detect a human energy field, "the claims of TT are groundless and that further professional use is unjustified" (Rosa et al.,

1998, p. 1005). Critics of the Rosa et al. (1998) study are quick to point up flaws in the study's experimental design and conclusions (Achterberg, 1998; Leskowitz, 1998). According to Leskowitz (1998), experimental bias was not addressed and perhaps somewhat exploited when a professional film crew videotaped the second round of trials for a television broadcast. Furthermore, Leskowitz (1998) suggests that the only reasonable conclusion of this study should have been that given this set of experimental conditions, the purported human energy field was not detectable. The authors had no basis to conclude from their data that TT is not effective in clinical situations because the intervention of TT as defined by Krieger (1979) was never administered.

Physical and occupational therapists considering the inclusion of TT into their practice should be aware of the promising, but limited research that has included subjects with diagnoses typically seen in rehabilitation. Given the difficulties that often arise in pain management for the elderly due to polypharmaceutical concerns and multi-biological changes, non-invasive and low-risk interventions for pain control is an area needing serious investigation. As professionals that address pain, impairment and dysfunction, physical and occupational therapists are probably well-suited to conduct research in modalities and approaches such as TT.

CONCLUSION

Physical and occupational therapists may not be qualified to diagnose or address all the problems facing older patients but an effort should be made to be aware of conditions or situations that may either positively or negatively affect the outcomes of a plan of care. Whether a patient informs a therapist of difficulty regulating one's blood sugar, or the patient receives a Reiki treatment once a week, therapists need to be able to appreciate how this information may or may not influence a therapeutic rehabilitation program and achievement of positive outcomes. On a broader and more ambitious spectrum, physical and occupational therapists may be well served to better understand the assumptions and theories of alternative healing approaches being sought by more and more Americans each year. As clinicians and researchers, physical and occupational therapists need to move forward in an effort to identify modalities, interventions and strategies that show promise in helping patients deal with and recover from pain, impairment, and dysfunction. At the same time, physical and occupational therapists need to investigate alternative and complementary approaches to health and well-being that may prevent or minimize pain, impairment, and dysfunction as people age.

This article's attempt to examine just a few alternative healing approaches and provide suggestions to physical and occupational therapists who may be considering incorporation of these approaches into their practices is just the beginning. Rehabilitation therapists interested in this area should consider scientific investigation of energy based therapies in search of evidence that these approaches are reasonable and valid. Only then will physical and occupational therapists be able to fully integrate these healing approaches into a traditional plan of care.

For further information:

Polarity Therapy
> American Polarity Therapy Association
> 2888 Bluff St., Suite 149
> Boulder, CO 80301
> 303-545-2080

Qigong
> National Qigong (Chi Kung) Assoc. * USA
> P.O. Box 540
> Ely, MN 55731
> 218-365-6330

> Qigong Association of America
> 2021 NW Grant Ave.
> Corvallis, OR 97330
> 541-752-6599

Reiki
> The Reiki Alliance
> P.O. Box 41
> Cataldo, ID 83810-1041
> 208-682-3535

> American Reiki Masters Association
> P.O. Box 130
> Lake City, FL 32056-0130
> 904-755-9638

Therapeutic Touch
   Nurse Healers–Professional Associates, International
   3760 South Highland Drive #429
   Salt Lake City, VT 84106

   Pumpkin Hollow Foundation
   RR #1, Box 135
   Craryville, NY 12521
   518-325-3583 or 518-325-7105

REFERENCES

Achterberg, J. (1998). Clearing the air in the therapeutic touch controversy. *Alternative Therapies in Health and Medicine, 4* (4), 100.

Ankun, K., Chongxing, W., Dinghai, X. & Yuesheng, W. (1991). Research on "anti-aging" effect on qigong. *Journal of Traditional Chinese Medicine, 11 (2), 153-158.*

Barnett, L. & Chambers, M. (1996). *Reiki energy medicine: Bringing healing touch into home, hospital, and hospice.* Rochester, VT: Healing Arts Press.

Becker, R.O. & Selden, G. (1985). *The body electric.* New York, NY: William Morrow and Company, Inc.

Benford, M.S., Talnagi, J., Burr Doss, D., Boosey, S. & Arnold, L.E. (1999). Gamma radiation fluctuations during alternative healing therapy. *Alternative Therapies in Health and Medicine, 5* (4), 51-56.

Capra, F. (1975). *The tao of physics.* Boston, MA: Shambhala Publications, Inc.

Claire, T. (1995). *Bodywork: What type of massage to get–and how to make the most of it.* New York, NY: William Morrow and Company, Inc.

Dong, P. & Esser, A. (1990). *Chi gong: The ancient Chinese way to health.* New York, NY: Marlowe and Company.

Dossey, B. M. (1997). Complementary and alternative therapies for our aging society. *Journal of Gerontological Nursing, 23* (9), 45-51.

Dossey, L. (1995). How should alternative therapies be evaluated? An examination of fundamentals. *Alternative Therapies in Health and Medicine, 1* (2), 6-10, 79-85.

Easter, A. (1997). The state of research on the effects of therapeutic touch. *Journal of Holistic Nursing, 15* (2), 158-175.

Eckes Peck, S. D. (1997). The effectiveness of therapeutic touch for decreasing pain in elders with degenerative arthritis. *Journal of Holistic Nursing, 15* (2), 176-198.

Eisenberg, D.M., Kessler, R.C., Foster, C., Norlock, F.E., Calkins, D.R. & Delbanco T.L. (1993). Unconventional medicine in the United States–prevalence, costs, and patterns of care. *New England Journal of Medicine, 328* (4), 246-252.

Gerber, R. (1988). *Vibrational medicine: New choices for healing ourselves.* (Rev. ed.). Santa Fe, NM: Bear and Company.

Gordon, A., Merenstein, J. H., D'Amico, F. & Hudgen, D. (1998). The effects of therapeutic touch on patients with osteoarthritis of the knee. *The Journal of Family Practice, 47* (4), 271-276.

Gordon, K. (1997). Acupuncture in the physical therapy clinic. In C.M. Davis (Ed.), *Complementary therapies in rehabilitation.* Thorofare, NJ: Slack, Inc.

Guccione, A.A. (1993). Implications of an aging population for rehabilitation: Demography, mortality, and morbidity in the elderly. In A.A. Guccione (Ed.), *Geriatric physical therapy.* St. Louis, MO: Mosby-Year Book, Inc.

Heidt, P. (1981). Effect of therapeutic touch on the anxiety level of hospitalized patients. *Nursing Research, 30 (1), 32-37.*

Helms, J. M. (1998). An overview of medical acupuncture. *Alternative Therapies in Health and Medicine, 4* (3), 35-45.

Horan, P. (1992). *Empowerment through Reiki* (2nd ed.). Wilmot, WI: Lotus Light.

Karagulla, S. & Kunz, D. (1989). *The chakras and the human energy field.* Wheaton, IL: Theosophical Publishing House.

Keller, E. & Bzdek, V. M. (1986). Effects of therapeutic touch on tension headache pain. *Nursing Research, 35* (2), 102-106.

Kitts, B. (1988). Polarity therapy. In F.M. Tappen (Ed.), *Healing massage techniques: Holistic, classic and emerging methods.* Englewood Cliffs, NJ: Prentice-Hall.

Krieger, D. (1979). *The therapeutic touch. How to use your hands to help or heal.* New York, NY: Simon and Schuster.

Krieger, D. (1993). *Accepting your power to heal: The personal practice of therapeutic touch.* Santa Fe, NM: Bear and Company, Inc.

Krieger, D. (1997). *Therapeutic touch inner workbook: Ventures in transpersonal healing.* Santa Fe, NM: Bear and Company, Inc.

Kunz, D. (1991). *The personal aura.* Wheaton, IL: Theosophical Publishing House.

Leskowitz, E. (1998). Un-debunking therapeutic touch. *Alternative Therapies in Health and Medicine, 4* (4), 101-102.

Luskin, F. M., Newell, K. A., Griffith, M., Holmes, M., Telles, S., Manasti, F. F., Pelletier, K. R. & Haskell, W. L. (1998). A review of mind-body therapies in the treatment of cardiovascular disease. Part 1: Implications for the elderly. *Alternative Therapies in Health and Medicine, 4* (3), 46-61.

Mansour, A. A., Beuche, M., Laing, G., Leis, A., & Nurse, J. (1999). A study to test the effectiveness of placebo Reiki standardization procedures developed for a planned Reiki efficacy study. *Journal of Alternative and Complementary Medicine, 5* (4), 153-164.

McCormack, G.L. & Galantino, M.L. (1997). Non-contact therapeutic touch. In C.M. Davis (Ed.), *Complementary therapies in rehabilitation.* Thorofare, NJ: Slack, Inc.

National Institutes of Health/National Center for Complementary and Alternative Medicine. (2000, Jan.). *What is CAM?/Classification of alternative medicine practices* (On-line). Available http://nccam.nih.gov/ncaam/fcp/classify/.

Olson, K. & Hanson, J. (1997). Using Reiki to manage pain: A preliminary report. *Cancer Prevention and Control, 1* (6), 108-113.

Olson, K. & Sneed, N. (1995). Anxiety and Therapeutic Touch. *Issues in Mental Health Nursing, 16,* 97-108.

Reid, D. (1994). *The complete book of Chinese health and healing*. Boston, MA: Shambhala Publications, Inc.

Rosa, L., Rosa, E., Sarner, L., & Barrett, S. (1998). A close look at Therapeutic Touch. *Journal of the American Medical Association, 279,* 1005-1010.

Ryu, H., Jun, C.D., Lee, B.S., Choi, B.M., Kim, H.M. & Chung, H.T. (1995). Effect of qigong training on proportions of t-lymphocyte subsets in human peripheral blood. *American Journal of Chinese Medicine, 23 (1), 27-36.*

Sancier, K.M. (1996). Medical applications of qigong. *Alternative Therapies in Health and Medicine, 2* (1), 40-46.

Sancier, K. (1996). Anti-aging benefits of qigong. *Journal of International Social Lifestyle Information Science, 14* (1), 12-20.

Scott, A. H. (1999). Wellness works: Community services health promotion groups led by occupational therapy students. *American Journal of Occupational Therapy, 53* (6), 566-574.

Selby, P. (1997). Subtle energy manipulation and physical therapy. In C.M. Davis (Ed.), *Complementary Therapies in Rehabilitation*. Thorofare, NJ: Slack, Inc.

Sharp, M. B. (1997). Polarity, reflexology and touch for health. In C. M. Davis (ed.), *Complementary Therapies in Rehabilitation*. Thorofare, NJ: Slack, Inc.

Sills, F. (1990). *The polarity process: Energy as a healing art*. Dorset, UK: Element Books.

Simington, J. A. & Laing, G. P. (1993). Effects of therapeutic touch on anxiety in the institutionalized elderly. *Clinical Nursing Research, 2* (4), 438-450.

Spence, J. E. & Olsen, M. A. (1997). Quantitative research of therapeutic touch. An integrative review of the literature 1985-1995. *Scandinavian Journal of Caring Science, 11* (3), 183-190. (From National Library of Medicine, 1999, NLM CIT. ID 98009773).

Turner, J.G., Clark, A. J., Gauthier, D.K. & Williams, M. (1998). The effect of therapeutic touch on pain and anxiety in burn patients. *Journal of Advanced Nursing, 28* (1), 10-28.

Veith, I. (1970). *The Yellow Emperor's Classic of Internal Medicine*. (I. Veith, Trans.). Berkeley, CA, University of California Press.

Winstead-Fry, P. & Kijek, J. (1999). An integrative review and meta-analysis of therapeutic touch research. *Alternative Therapies in Health and Medicine, 5* (6), 58-67.

Wolf, S.L., Barnhart, H. X., Ellison, G. L. & Coogler, C. E. (1997). The effect of Tai Chi Quan and computerized balance training on postural stability in older subjects. Atlanta FICSIT Frailty and Injuries: Cooperative studies on intervention techniques. *Physical Therapy, 77* (4), 371-381.

Wu, W., Bandilla, E., Ciccone, D.S., Yang, J., Cheng, S.S., Carner, N., Wu, Y. & Shen, R. (1999). Effects of qigong on late-stage complex regional pain syndrome. *Alternative Therapies in Health and Medicine, 5* (1), 45-54.

Mental Rehearsal
as a Complementary Treatment
in Geriatric Rehabilitation

Nancy T. Fell, PT, MHS, NCS
Craig A. Wrisberg, PhD

SUMMARY. The challenge of geriatric rehabilitation continues to grow with decreasing Medicare reimbursement and societal access to therapy. Occupational and physical therapists must be proactive in developing strategies that optimize therapy outcomes for patients. Mental rehearsal is a complementary treatment technique that should be considered for facilitation of motor skill acquisition. This technique has been used extensively in sport, music, and dance performance. While it is not a viable substitute for physical practice, it most certainly can be helpful in motor learning enhancement. The purpose of this article is to provide an overview of mental rehearsal: describe mental rehearsal, review the available research on the topic, consider possible mechanisms of action, and suggest its application to the geriatric patient population. *[Article copies available for a fee from The Haworth Document Delivery Service: 1-800- 342-9678. E-mail address: <getinfo@haworthpressinc.com> Website: <http:// www.HaworthPress. com> © 2001 by The Haworth Press, Inc. All rights reserved.]*

Nancy T. Fell is Assistant Professor of Physical Therapy, University of Tennessee at Chattanooga, 615 McCallie Avenue, Chattanooga, TN 37403.

Craig A. Wrisberg is Professor of Sport Psychology, University of Tennessee, Knoxville, 1914 Andy Holt Avenue, Knoxville, TN 37996-2700.

[Haworth co-indexing entry note]: "Mental Rehearsal as a Complementary Treatment in Geriatric Rehabilitation." Fell, Nancy T., and Craig A. Wrisberg. Co-published simultaneously in *Physical & Occupational Therapy in Geriatrics* (The Haworth Press, Inc.) Vol. 18, Number 4, 2001, pp. 51-63; and: *Complementary Therapies in Geriatric Practice: Selected Topics* (ed: Ann Burkhardt, and Jodi Carlson) The Haworth Press, Inc., 2001, pp. 51-63. Single or multiple copies of this article are available for a fee from The Haworth Document Delivery Service [1-800-342-9678, 9:00 a.m. - 5:00 p.m. (EST). E-mail address: getinfo@haworthpressinc.com].

KEYWORDS. Mental rehearsal, imagery, motor skill acquisition, occupational therapy, physical therapy, geriatric rehabilitation, alternative therapy

INTRODUCTION

Occupational and physical therapists commonly work with patients to facilitate their learning of motor activities, whether for the fine-tuning of coordinated movements or the acquisition of new, compensatory strategies. Historically, the focus of physical rehabilitation has been on physical practice with an emphasis on specificity of exercise in randomly-structured practice sessions. In other domains (e.g., athletics, performing arts, dance), performers often supplement physical training with mental rehearsal in order to enhance their skill levels.

Mental rehearsal is referred to by many names in the scientific literature. Some of these include visualization, mental practice, mental imagery, imaginary practice, conceptualizing, and covert rehearsal. While some authors attempt to distinguish the meanings of these terms (Schmidt & Wrisberg, 2000), more often the labels have been used interchangeably (Richardson, 1967a, 1967b; Feltz & Landers, 1983; Sheikh & Korn, 1994). For the purposes of this article, mental rehearsal (MR) is defined as the mental or cognitive imagining of some aspect of the performance of a task or skill in the absence of any associated overt physical actions. Schmidt and Lee (1999) have observed that MR can produce large positive results and transfer improved skill to the performance of an actual physical task. For the most part, however, it appears that rehabilitation professionals have not considered the benefits of such an approach in lieu of or as an adjunct to physical practice. Therefore, the purpose of this article is to present an overview of the concept of MR and suggest possible applications of this type of adjunct therapy within the domain of geriatric occupational and physical therapy.

A DIFFERENT PARADIGM

The premise that MR is a potentially beneficial form of practice for improving physical performance is deeply embedded in the holistic notion of a mind-body connection. Unfortunately, the currently accepted medical model of scientific research seems to circumvent this relationship. The traditional Western approach to medicine and the scientific method originated in the 17th century and was significantly influenced by the thinking of Rene Descartes, Isaac Newton, and John Dewey. Newtonian-Cartesian physics is based primarily on the mechanical laws of cause and effect and the search for that which is "real" by the proof or disproof of hypotheses. The scientific method has also been described as discovery through reductionism: Scientists attempt to reduce the influence of any interfering variables–including those of chance or luck–to, as rigorously as possible, determine the effect of the treatment variable (Kuhn, 1979). It is clear that traditional Western medicine treats infectious disease, acute illness, and trauma more effectively than any other health care system in the world. However, there are unexplained phenomena that exist which the current Western model largely ignores (Davis, 1997). Perhaps the best medical example of such a phenomenon is the placebo effect. Ironically, this effect may be the cornerstone of a new and improved understanding of the mind-body connection and physical healing (Rossi, 1986).

Traditional scientific methodology strives to separate the body from the mind and emphasizes only those phenomena that can be physically observed. Yet even C. Everett Koop, former United States Surgeon General, states that appropriate responses to crises in modern medicine lie in the development of alternative medicine (Koop, 1996). It is interesting to note that in 1990, one third of the population of the United States was estimated to have used some form of alternative therapy, and it is likely that today the percentage is far higher (Gordon, 1998). According to the World Health Organization, 80 percent of all people worldwide use these "alternatives" as their form of primary care (Gordon, 1998). The former Surgeon General's stance and the evolving curiosity of still other traditional physicians have been impacted further by discoveries emanating from a special area of Western medical research, psychoneuroimmunology.

In recent years, psychoneuroimmunology researchers have identified a continuous dialogue between the mind, nervous, and immune systems, which suggests that emotions can affect the immune system in both positive and negative ways. More specifically, two pathways of communication that have been identified are the autonomic nervous system (sympathetic and parasympathetic) and the immune system of neurotransmitters and neuropeptides (Davis, 1996). Interactions between the mind and these two systems have been shown to exist in diseases such as HIV, cancer, and arthritis (Gorman & Kertzner, 1991). Such research makes it increasingly difficult to ignore the mind-body connection in the diagnosis and treatment of disorders.

Holism's theoretical base emphasizes the importance of the interaction of energy, people, and matter to the larger whole, which is always more than the sum of the parts (Davis, 1997). The biological reality of the human being is both the unseen mind and the material body, and all of the cells of the body are interconnected with the mind while the mind is very much interconnected with each cell in the body. The lay-terminology of "holistic, complementary, unconventional, and alternative" generally refers to forms of healing that emerged from traditional Native American and Eastern medicine and wellness notions that have been effectively utilized for thousands of years. Holism is, from a Western perspective, based on the theories of quantum physics as developed by Einstein, Bohm, and others (Davis, 1997). This approach carries the assumption that all individuals are different and that the manifestations of disease depend on the unique characteristics of the individual patient. Alternative health care practitioners generally place greater emphasis on the validity of each individual therapeutic experience. Whatever the case may be, it appears that further research is needed, incorporating both qualitative and quantitative methodologies, to further substantiate the mind-body connection.

SUPPORT FOR MENTAL REHEARSAL

There is a significant body of athletic research that supports the benefits of MR for physical performance. However, it is important to consider the many nuances involved in the designs used in different studies. One conclusion that appears warranted is that physical practice has a greater effect on motor performance than does MR, which in turn is better than no practice at all (Corbin, 1972; Feltz & Landers, 1983; Richardson, 1967a, 1967b). This conclusion is based on the results of studies that have primarily examined three types of practice conditions: physical rehearsal, MR, and no rehearsal (control). In one of the earliest studies, Sackett (1934) found that physical practice was superior to mental practice, but that mental practice was more effective in improving performance than no practice. Vandall, Davis, and Clugston (1943) investigated the effects of physical and mental practice on dart throwing and found that MR improved performance almost as much as physical practice.

Early reviews of the MR literature suggested that a combination of MR and physical practice is superior to either MR or physical practice alone (Richardson, 1967a, 1967b; Weinberg, 1982). More recent reviews (e.g., Feltz, Landers, & Becker, 1988) suggest that if the total number of practice trials (mental and/or physical) are equated, a combination of MR and physical practice (involving relatively fewer physical trials) is not more effective than physical practice alone.

Recently, Hall, Schmidt, Durand, and Buckolz (1994) found that the use of MR as a supplement to physical practice, rather than as a replacement for a portion of physical practice, results in improved performance (as compared to physical practice alone). In this study, an MR program was incorporated into the athlete's overall training program without reducing the total amount of physical practice time. Using a similar approach, Blair, Hall, and Leyshon (1993) compared the performance of soccer players who were assigned to a physical practice group and a physical practice plus MR group. The results revealed that the combined practice group improved significantly more than the group engaging in physical practice alone. Therefore, the authors suggested that MR be used as an adjunct to physical practice in order to facilitate performance.

Other considerations in the sport literature on MR include the skill level of the participant and the type of skill being performed or learned. Feltz and Landers (1983) conducted a meta-analysis of 60 MR studies and found that, regardless of the skill level of participants, mental practice was more effective for tasks that contained a greater number of cognitive-symbolic components than for tasks that were more motoric in nature. There is also considerable evidence that, for less experienced individuals, alternating mental practice with physical practice is an effective strategy for improving motor performance and learning (Etnier & Landers, 1996; Gabriele, Hall, & Lee, 1989; McBride & Rothstein, 1979).

Hall (1985) suggests that researchers consider three variables when studying the effects of MR, or more specifically mental imagery, on motor performance and learning. These are the imagery ability of the participant, the type of task being performed, and the imagery instructions given to participants. Smith (1987) has also suggested that researchers and practitioners consider the preferred imagery perspective of participants. Some individuals prefer an internal perspective (e.g., seeing and feeling the task exactly the way they would if they were physically performing it). Other people prefer an external imagery perspective (e.g., seeing themselves performing the task as if they were a spectator).

THEORIES FOR MENTAL REHEARSAL

While outcome measures seem to support the notion that MR is an effective tool for improving physical performance, less is known about the mechanisms producing these effects. How can physical motor learning be enhanced by MR in the absence of movement? How can motor learning occur as the result of a type of rehearsal in which there is neither movement nor movement-produced feedback?

Some theories suggest that mental rehearsal exerts an influence on several areas of the neuromuscular system. Washburn (1916) proposed one of the first hypotheses to explain the mechanisms underlying the MR effect. She contended that slight muscle movements were made when a person imagined himself/herself engaged in physical activity. These "movements" were presumed to be identical to the movements of the actual activity, except of much smaller magnitudes. Later, Jacobson (1932) produced support for this hypothesis by using electromyography (EMG) and observing that minute muscle contractions during MR occurred only in the muscles that were involved in the imagined activity. As a result, Jacobson proposed the psychoneuromuscular theory for MR. This theory holds that during the imaging of an activity, the brain sends out low levels of impulses that travel along the nerves to the muscles that produce the imagined movement. These impulses are presumed to be similar to those that would be emitted during actual physical performance of the activity, but are so slight as to be only detectable with EMG (Janssen & Sheikh, 1994).

While some researchers (Bird, 1984; Freeman, 1933; Suinn, 1972) have provided experimental and clinical support for Jacobson's theory, others have been unable to replicate similar EMG patterns for imagined and real movement, suggesting that muscle activation may not be exactly the same for both mental and physical practice. Feltz and Landers (1983) and Hecker and Kaczor (1988) have pointed out that some of the early research lacked appropriate methodological precision, and, in several cases (e.g., Shaw, 1938), researchers reported increased muscle action potentials that occurred throughout a broader section of the body rather than in task-specific muscle groups whenever participants imaged a particular movement.

Another early theory that was advanced to explain the beneficial effects of MR was the symbolic learning theory of Sackett (1934). According to Sackett, MR facilitated learning of a motor skill by the symbolic coding of movement patterns in the central nervous system (CNS). It was, therefore, predicted that tasks possessing a greater number of cognitive elements benefited relatively more from MR. Sackett also contended that symbolic learning was important only during the very early stages of motor learning (verbal-cognitive stage) when individuals were trying to get a general idea of the desired movement pattern. However, more recent scholars have discovered that MR can be important at all stages of practice depending upon the nature of the task (Magill, 1998). For example, MR would assist performers at all skill levels in sports like gymnastics and golf in focusing their attention on task-relevant cues that are necessary for subsequent physical performance (Schmidt & Wrisberg, 2000; Wrisberg & Ragsdale, 1979).

In more recent years, a third theory has been proposed by Lang (1977), who contends that MR becomes more important after an individual has participated in sufficient physical practice to create an internal image of the movement. Lang's bioinformational theory holds that, during MR, the internal image is activated, rehearsed, and reinforced, leading to improved performance once physical activity is resumed. McKay (1981) has further suggested that muscle units are "primed" for action during MR and that the extent to which this priming benefits subsequent physical performance depends on the previous amount of physical practice or experience the person has with the task. Such a view supports the notion that high-performance athletes benefit considerably more from mental imagery than do novice performers (Vealey & Greenleaf, 1998).

The bioinformational theory has neuroanatomical support as well. A close functional equivalence between motor imagery and motor preparation for physical performance is suggested by the positive effects of imagining motor learning, the similarity between the neural structures involved, and the similar physiological correlates observed in both imaging and preparing (Jeannerod, 1994). Based on the premise that MR improves motor performance and is accompanied by heightened CNS activity in healthy individuals, Weiss and colleagues (1994) studied brain activation during MR in stroke patients. Using electroencephalography (EEG), these researchers observed significant decreases of theta, alpha, as well as beta-1 brain waves during MR in comparison to a control period of rest only. Such changes are similar to those obtained for healthy individuals. Decreases in theta and alpha waves during MR may indicate an activation of the sensorimotor cortex which, in accordance with the hypothesis of internal feedback mechanisms, is a necessary prerequisite for motor learning.

IMPLICATIONS FOR GERIATRIC REHABILITATION

In addition to the available research showing improvements in motor skill acquisition with MR, there is some evidence that MR improves other physical performance variables as well. More specifically, strength and endurance have been shown to improve when physical practice is coupled with MR (Cornwall, Buscato, & Barry, 1991; Yue & Cole, 1992). While the vast majority of research examining the effects of MR has involved laboratory models using discrete motor or sports-related tasks, a few studies have addressed the use of MR with more functionally applied tasks. Ulich (1967) studied typewriting speed and accuracy, peg hole test manual dexterity and speed, and riveting speed and sequencing. The results of this study support the use of MR to facilitate performance improvements. Interestingly, the nursing profession has applied MR during the learning of psychomotor tasks required in their entry-level curriculum. Bucher (1993) and Doheny (1993) found that MR combined with physical practice enhanced nursing students' capability of donning and doffing sterile gloves and giving an intramuscular injection. Additionally, researchers have demonstrated that musical performance has been enhanced through the combination of MR and physical practice (Coffman, 1990; Theiler & Lippman, 1995).

When considering the application of MR to the elderly population, thought must be given to age-related changes in musculoskeletal and neurological systems. For example, Briggs, Raz, and Marks (1999) investigated the age-related slowing of information processing in mental imagery tasks and found that age was associated with prolongation of response time. Moreover, older individuals benefited relatively less from MR as the information to be processed increased in complexity. These researchers concluded that the slowing of information processing and reduction in accuracy of older individuals was mediated by declines in working memory rather than by decreases in sensorimotor speed. However, Dror and Kosslyn (1994) compared the performance of young and elderly adults on four visual mental imagery tasks–rotation, activation, composition, and scanning–and found that, while there was a slowing with age, individual imaging processes appeared to be selectively affected by aging.

The effect of MR on elders' motor skill acquisition has received little experimental attention to date. Surburg (1976) randomly assigned 140 participants representing two elder age groups (65-79 and 80-100) to one of four practice conditions: physical practice, one-half physical practice, physical-mental practice, or a control group with no practice.

Individuals were initially tested on a pursuit rotor task, then practiced the task (according to their respective conditions of group assignment), then were retested, and then were retested 8 weeks later. The results revealed that, for both age groups, the combination of physical and mental practice was as effective as either of the other two types of physical practice alone.

Fansler, Poff, and Shepard (1985) were the first therapists to apply the concepts of MR to clinical research in the physical therapy profession and to publish their research. In this study, 12 female elders utilized ideokinetic facilitation, a type of MR, in an effort to enhance physical performance of balance tasks. Following training, an experimental group that participated in a combination of mental and physical practice demonstrated significant improvements in performance. However, these improvements were not significantly greater than those of control groups participating in physical practice and relaxation or in physical practice and listening to nonsense tapes. While the results of this study were inconclusive, the authors suggested that, "Mental practice of a physical task can improve performance and may be of use to the physical therapy clinician" (p. 1332). Warner and McNeill (1988) further addressed the issue of MR with an article published in *Physical Therapy* presenting a review of the pertinent literature and suggesting the feasibility of MR as an adjunctive technique for rehabilitation. Occupational and physical therapists, however, appear to have not adequately considered the potential benefits of MR in physical rehabilitation.

CONCLUSION

The overwhelming evidence from a number of different performance domains reveals that physical practice is superior to MR in facilitating the learning of motor skills. However, it has also been shown that MR is superior to no practice in many situations (Feltz & Landers, 1983). This evidence suggests that MR is a potentially effective technique for patients whose physical activity is restricted or whose physical practice is limited or prohibited (Warner & McNeill, 1988). In the rehabilitation professions, particularly those dealing with elder adults, there are numerous instances in which physical practice is contraindicated or must be provided only with extreme caution. For many elders, a safe environment, necessary equipment, or the presence of a person to assist in physical exercise may not always be available. There are also times when elders' physical practice must be limited because of cardiac or pulmonary complications. For the deconditioned older adult, fatigue may severely inhibit the rehabilitative process following injury or surgery. In such instances, MR as an adjunct to physical practice would seem logical. Moreover, MR might be beneficial in minimizing functional losses related to immobilization and facilitating the rehabilitation process.

Recently, managed care has decreased the available number and length of therapy visits for many patients. Often, elderly patients spend less time engaging in the physical practice of functional tasks under the supervision of a therapist. It would appear that, more than ever, MR should be considered as a potential adjunct to conventional therapy.

While resourceful therapists may be able to find ways to intertwine the two rehearsal modes of physical practice and MR to promote maximal performance gains, they should do so only after appropriate training. Both the experimental and anecdotal evidence clearly indicates that imagery techniques can be a valuable tool in improving physical performance; however, they must be applied with care. Just as it is difficult to relearn a task when it has been physically learned incorrectly, it is also difficult to physically relearn a task once it has been mentally practiced incorrectly (Sheikh & Korn, 1994). The best resources for learning general application guidelines in MR continue to be basic sport psychology texts. Some of the most practical include *Psyching for Sport: Mental Training for Athletes* (Orlick, 1986) and *Applied Sport Psychology: Personal Growth to Peak Performance* (Williams, 1997). Both are available through major booksellers. Mental rehearsal information on the Internet is growing. While websites for general overview and guidelines are limited (e.g., <http://www.enhanced-performance.com/nideffer/articles/Poland.html>), there are many sites with sport-specific information on MR application (e.g., <http://mindplusmuscle.com/html/mental_rehearsal.html>, <http://www.psychinnovations.com> and <http://www.onthenet.com.au/~rjudson/imagery.htm>).

As more and more therapists learn the techniques of MR and examine their effectiveness in the rehabilitation setting, the amount of evidence in support of its use for the elderly should also increase. Research is needed to identify whether MR will be efficient and effective in rehabilitation. Additionally, research must determine if there are specific situations or settings where MR is more or less effective. Perhaps, in time, MR will become less of an alternative or adjunct therapy technique and become a technique that is an obvious and natural component of every rehabilitation program.

REFERENCES

Bird, E. (1984). EMG Quantification of Mental Rehearsal. *Perceptual and Motor Skills*, 59, 899-906.

Blair, A.M., Hall, X., & Leyshon, X. (1993). Imagery Effects on the Performance of Skilled and Novice Soccer Players. *Journal of Sport Sciences*, 11, 95-101.

Briggs, S.D., Raz, N., & Marks, W. (1999). *Psychology of Aging*, 14, 427-35.

Bucher, L. (1993). The Effects of Imagery Abilities and Mental Rehearsal on Learning a Nursing Skill. *Journal of Nursing Education*, 32, 318-24.

Coffman, D.D. (1990). Effects of Mental Practice, Physical Practice, and Knowledge of Results on Piano Performance. *Journal of Research in Music Education*, 38, 187-96.

Corbin, C.B. (1972). Mental Practice. In W.P. Morgan (Ed.), *Ergogenic Aids and Muscular Performance*. New York, NY: Academic Press.

Cornwall, M.W., Buscato, M.P. & Barry, S. (1991). Effect of Mental Practice on Isometric Muscular Strength. *Journal of Orthopaedic and Sports Physical Therapy*, 13, 231-4.

Davis, C.M. (1996). Psychosocial Aspects of Aging. In C.B. Lewis (Ed.), *Aging the Health Care Challenge*, (3rd ed.), (p. 40). Philadelphia, PA: F.A. Davis Company.

Davis, C.M. (1997). Introduction and Psychoneuroimmunology: The Bridge to the Coexistence of Two Paradigms. In C.M. Davis (Ed.), *Complementary Therapies in Rehabilitation* (pp. 1-15). Thorofare, NJ: Slack Incorporated.

Dohney, M.O. (1993). Mental Practice: An Alternative Approach to Teaching Motor Skills. *Journal of Nursing Education*, 32, 260-4.

Dror, I.E. & Kosslyn, S.M. (1994). Mental Imagery and Aging. *Psychology of Aging*, 9, 90-102.

Etnier, J. & Landers, D.M. (1996). The Influence of Procedural Variables on the Efficacy of Mental Practice. *The Sport Psychologist*, 10, 48-57.

Fansler, C.L., Poff, C.L., & Shepard, K.F. (1985). Effects of Mental Practice on Balance in Elderly Women. *Physical Therapy*, 65, 1332-7.

Feltz, D. & Landers, D. (1983). The Effects of Mental Practice on Motor Skill Learning and Performance: A Meta-analysis. *Journal of Sport Psychology*, 5, 25-57.

Feltz, D.L., Landers, D.M., & Becker, B.J. (1988). A Revised Meta-analysis of the Mental Practice Literature on Motor Skill Learning. In D. Druckman & J. Swets (Eds.), *Enhancing Human Performance: Issues, Theories, and Techniques* (pp. 1-65). Washington, DC: National Academy Press.

Freeman, G.L. (1933). The Facilitation and Inhibitory Effect of Muscular Tension Upon Performance. *American Journal of Psychology*, 45, 17-52.

Gabriele, T., Hall, C.R. & Lee, T.D. (1989). Cognition in Motor Learning: Imagery Effects on Contextual Interference. *Human Movement Science*, 8, 227-45.

Gordon, J. (1998) Changing How We Define Medicine. *Center for Mind-Body Medicine*. <www.healthy.net/othersites/mindbody/mblibrary/oamreport.htm>.

Gorman, J.M. & Kertzner, R.M. (1991). *Psychoimmunology*. Washington, D.C.: American Psychiatric Press.

Hall, C.R. (1985). Individual Differences in the Mental Practice and Imagery of Motor Skill Performance. *Canadian Journal of Applied Sport Science*, 10, 17S-21S.

Hall, C., Schmidt, D., Durand, M.C., & Buckolz, E. (1994). Imagery and Motor Skills Acquisition. In A.A. Sheikh & E.R. Korn (Eds.), *Imagery in Sports and Physical Performance* (pp. 122-123). Amityville, NY: Baywood Publishing.

Hecker, J.E. & Kaczor, L.M. (1988). Application of Imagery Theory to Sport Psychology: Some Preliminary Findings. *Journal of Sport Psychology*, 10, 363-73.

Jacobson, E. (1932). Electrophysiology of Mental Activities. *American Journal of Psychology*, 44, 677-94.

Janssen, J.J. & Sheikh, A.A. (1994). Enhancing Athletic Performance Through Imagery: An Overview. In A.A. Sheikh & E.R. Korn (Eds.), *Imagery in Sports and Physical Performance* (pp. 1-22). Amityville, NY: Baywood Publishing Company.

Jeannerod, M. (1994). The Representing Brain: Neural Correlates of Motor Intention and Imagery. *Behavioral and Brain Sciences*, 17, 187-245.

Koop, C.E. (1996). Foreword–the Art and Science of Medicine. In M.S. Micozzi (Ed.), *Fundamentals of Complementary and Alternative Medicine*. New York, NY: Churchill Livingstone.

Kuhn, T. S. (1979). *Structure of Scientific Revolutions*. Chicago, IL: University of Chicago Press.

Lang, P.J. (1977). Imagery in Therapy: An Information Processing Analysis of Fear. *Behavior Therapy*, 8, 862-86.

MacKay, D.G. (1981). The Problem of Rehearsal or Mental Practice. *Journal of Motor Behavior*, 13, 274-85.

Magill, R.A. (1998). *Motor Learning: Concepts and Applications*. (5th ed.). Dubuque, IA: Brown.

McBride, E. & Rothstein, A. (1979). Mental and Physical Practice and the Learning and Retention of Open and Closed Skills. *Perceptual and Motor Skills*, 49, 359-65.

Orlick, T. (1986). *Psyching for Sport: Mental Training for Athletes*. Champaign, IL: Human Kinetics.

Richardson, A. (1967a). Mental Practice: A Review and Discussion, Part I. *Research Quarterly*, 38, 95-107.

Richardson, A. (1967b). Mental Practice: A Review and Discussion, Part II. *Research Quarterly*, 38, 263-73.

Rossi, E.R. (1986). *The Psychobiology of Mind-Body Healing*. New York, NY: W.W. Norton and Company.

Sackett, R.S. (1934). The Influences of Symbolic Rehearsal Upon the Retention of a Maze Habit. *Journal of General Psychology*, 10, 376-95.

Schmidt, R.A. & Lee, T.D. (1999). *Motor Control and Learning: A Behavioral Emphasis*. (3rd ed.). Champaign, IL: Human Kinetics.

Schmidt, R.A. & Wrisberg, C.A. (2000). *Motor Learning and Performance*. (2nd ed.). Champaign, IL: Human Kinetics.

Shaw, W. (1938). The Distribution of Muscle Action Potentials During Imaging. *The Psychological Record*, 2, 195-216.

Sheikh, A.A. & Korn, E.R. (1994). *Imagery in Sports and Physical Performance*. Amityville, NY: Baywood Publishing.

Smith, D. (1987). Conditions that Facilitate the Development of Sport Imagery Training. *The Sport Psychologist*, 1, 237-247.

Suinn, R.M. (1972). Behavioral Rehearsal Training for Ski Racers. *Behavior Therapy*, 3, 519.

Surburg, P.R. (1976). Aging and Effect of Physical-Mental Practice upon Acquisition and Retention of a Motor Skill. *Journal of Gerontology*, 31, 64-7.

Theiler, A.M. & Lippman, L.G. (1995). Effects of Mental Practice and Modeling on Guitar and Vocal Performance. *Journal of General Psychology*, 122, 329-343.

Ulich, E. (1967). Some Experiments on the Function of Mental Training in the Acquisition of Motor Skills. *Ergonomics*, 10, 411-9.

Vandall, R.A., Davis, R.A., & Clugston, H.A. (1943). The Function of Mental Practice in the Acquisition of Motor Skills. *Journal of General Psychology*, 29, 243-50.

Vealey, R.S. & Greenleaf, C.A. (1998). Seeing Is Believing: Understanding and Using Imagery in Sport. In J.M. Williams (Ed.), *Applied Sport Psychology: Personal Growth to Peak Performance* (pp. 237-260). Mountain View, CA: Mayfield.

Warner, L. & McNeill, M.E. (1988). Mental Imagery and Its Potential for Physical Therapy. *Physical Therapy*, 68, 516-21.

Washburn, F.F. (1916). *Movement and Mental Imagery*. Boston, MA: Houghton.

Weinberg, R.S. (1982). The Relationship between Mental Preparation Strategies and Motor Performance: A Review and Critique. *Quest*, 33, 195-213.

Weiss, T., Hansen, E., Beyer, L., Conradi, M.L., Merten, F., Nichelmann, C., Rost, R. & Zippel, C. (1994). Activation Processes During Mental Practice in Stroke Patients. *International Journal of Psychophysiology*, 17, 91-100.

Williams, J.M. (1997). *Applied Sport Psychology: Personal Growth to Peak Performance*. (3rd ed.). Mountain View, CA: Mayfield Publishing Company.

Wrisberg, C.A. & Ragsdale, M.R. (1979). Cognitive Demand and Practice Level: Factors in the Mental Rehearsal of Motor Skills. *Journal of Human Movement Studies*, 5, 201-8.

Yue, G. & Cole, K.J. (1992). Strength Increases from the Motor Program: Comparison of Training with Maximal Voluntary and Imagined Muscle Contractions. *Journal of Neurophysiology*, 67, 1114-23.

Addressing Spirituality and Religious Life in Occupational Therapy Practice

Joanne E. Farrar, MSc, OTR/L

SUMMARY. Health care practitioners are urged by third party payers to deliver meaningful, effective, and enduring therapy with minimal treatment time and staff. Treatment plans designed to enliven the spirit may excite the client to internalize treatment interventions, resulting in improved outcomes.

Physicians, psychiatrists, and nurses are being trained in the therapeutic use of spirituality, religion, and complementary medicine to maximize wellness. A survey of Canadian and U.S. occupational therapists was conducted to determine whether occupational therapists are addressing spirituality and religion in practice. Data was collected which identifies practical problems occupational therapists encounter. The majority of respondents felt spirituality appropriate for occupational therapy practice; one third stated religion is appropriate for treatment planning, but most respondents were unsure how to do so. Respondents identified information needed to address the client's spirituality or religion in occupational therapy practice. *[Article copies available for a fee from The Haworth Document Delivery Service: 1-800-342-9678. E-mail address: <getinfo@ haworthpressinc.com> Website: <http://www.HaworthPress.com> © 2001 by The Haworth Press, Inc. All rights reserved.]*

KEYWORDS. Spirituality, religion, wellness, mind and body connection, psychoneuroimmunology, spiritual crisis

---

Joanne E. Farrar is an Occupational Therapist with Integrated Health Services of New Hampshire at Claremont, P.O. Box 301, Canaan, NH 03741.

[Haworth co-indexing entry note]: "Addressing Spirituality and Religious Life in Occupational Therapy Practice." Farrar, Joanne E. Co-published simultaneously in *Physical & Occupational Therapy in Geriatrics* (The Haworth Press, Inc.) Vol. 18, Number 4, 2001, pp. 65-85; and: *Complementary Therapies in Geriatric Practice: Selected Topics* (ed: Ann Burkhardt, and Jodi Carlson) The Haworth Press, Inc., 2001, pp. 65-85. Single or multiple copies of this article are available for a fee from The Haworth Document Delivery Service [1-800-342-9678, 9:00 a.m. - 5:00 p.m. (EST). E-mail address: getinfo@haworthpressinc.com].

In 1910, the founders of occupational therapy believed the client's mind, body and spirit must be considered when designing and adapting therapeutic activities (Quiroga, 1995). Despite occupational therapists' successful outcomes, medical doctors required scientific proof for treatment interventions. In order to enhance the professional status of occupational therapy, therapists acquiesced to the model of medical science as originally defined by Descartes, and religion was excluded from the realm of occupational therapy practice (Quiroga, 1995). Psychoneuroimmunology research now demonstrates a biological model by which emotions affect cell physiology. As a result, occupational therapists addressing the whole person (body, mind, and spirit) may offer more comprehensive interventions than therapists who address only physical or psychological needs of the client.

LITERATURE REVIEW

Researchers have demonstrated a biological basis for the mind-body connection (Pert, 1993; Cousins, 1989; Melnechuk, 1988), and Western medicine is beginning to incorporate Eastern practices to optimize medical outcome (Wirth, 1993; Kabat-Zin, 1990; Benson & Klipper, 1975; Benson & Proctor, 1985, 1987; Benson, 1996; McCormack, 1992). Occupational therapists address the physical and psychological aspects of the client's health, and, in pragmatic terms, the client's spirit is addressed when meaningful activity is the focus of occupational therapy practice (Urbanowsky, 1997).

Psychoneuroimmunology demonstrates that the body and mind are inextricably connected. At the cellular level, bidirectional physical links have been discovered between emotions and attitudes, the central nervous system, and the immune system. Neuropeptides are the biochemical equivalent of emotions and are the bridge between body and mind; these chemicals control the migration of monocytes in healing and disease (Pert, 1993). Psychoneuroimmunology research shows that positive thoughts enhance the healing process and quality of life, and negative thoughts can result in physical illness and disease (Cousins, 1989; Gutterman, 1990).

The mind-body connection is the basis for the relationship between spirituality, faith, and wellness. Dr. Herbert Benson's research at Harvard Medical School during the past twenty-five years has described the relaxation response as the physiological benefits of mind-body interactions (Benson & Klipper, 1975). Stress-related diseases tend to be treated effectively by eliciting the relaxation response (Benson & Proctor, 1985; Benson & Proctor, 1987). Medical research confirms the traditional notion that people who practice their chosen religion tend to be healthier than those without this resource (Koenig, 1994; Koenig, 1995; Koenig, Kvale, & Ferrel, 1988; Oleckno, 1991).

Occupational therapy literature reflects therapists' uncertainty as to whether the client's spirit and religion are appropriate to address in practice (Burkhardt, 1997; Engquist, Short-DeGraff, Gliner, & Oltjenbruns, 1997; Stahl, 1994). Why are therapists uncertain about addressing spirituality in occupational therapy practice? Is the client's spirituality or religion relevant to occupational therapy practice? What do occupational therapists want to know about addressing spirituality and religion in practice?

The Canadian Association of Occupational Therapy (CAOT) and the Department of National Health and Welfare, Canada, developed a book of guidelines to assist therapists with spirituality and religion from initial evaluation through discharge planning (CAOT, 1991, p. 3). The philosophical basis of the guidelines is that the client's spirituality is the foundation of meaningful activity.

Blain and Townsend (1993) conducted a survey of Canadian occupational therapists to reassess the guidelines' practical use in occupational therapy practice. The Canadian respondents were about equally divided between feeling that spirituality is complicated yet appropriate for occupational therapy treatment, and the other half felt spirituality should be addressed by clergy.

Engquist et al. (1997) surveyed U.S. occupational therapists' beliefs regarding spirituality and therapy. While the respondents felt spirituality important personally and for clients' health and rehabilitation, less than half felt spirituality appropriate for occupational therapy practice. The majority felt that occupational therapists are not adequately trained to address spirituality. The authors suggested the response rate and results may have been affected by their choosing not to operationally define spirituality for the respondents. Taylor et al. (2000) extended Engquist et al.'s research to determine whether the therapist's own views regarding religiousness and spirituality affected the definition of spirituality, and, therefore, affected clinical reasoning regarding whether and how to address spirituality in occupational therapy practice

Rosenfeld wrote that spirituality is "meaning-making through purposeful activity" (2000, p. 17) and used the term "spiritual agent modality" for restoring function. When a client experiences a personal loss in functional capacity, rehabilitation offers the client an opportunity to resume personally meaningful daily activity. Rosenfeld described 11 prayer-crafting steps to adapt for the specific needs of this population (2000).

METHOD

After extensive literature review, the author was unable to find an existing instrument with which to conduct this research. Hence a survey was designed in conjunction with advisors Helen Smith and Diana Bailey at Tufts University. Survey questions were written to distinguish spirituality from religion to clarify therapists' opinions regarding these controversial topics (M. Pizzi, personal communication, December 1994). The pilot test of six occupational therapists was administered at *Youville Hospital and Rehabilitation Center* in Cambridge, MA, and appropriate survey modifications were made to enhance clarity. The number of pilot subjects was small and limited to U.S. therapists for reasons of time and resources. Pilot subjects' profiles generally corresponded with the survey subjects'. Pilot subjects' comments were used to make minor revisions to clarify questions.

The subjects were 200 Canadian and 210 United States occupational therapists randomly chosen from the membership of CAOT and AOTA. Data was collected in the fall of 1995. Data was accepted for all respondents who were currently employed as occupational therapists; no data was obtained from occupational therapy assistants. The author selected Canadian occupational therapists as research subjects in addition to U.S. occupational therapists because the researcher felt the Canadian experience addressing spirituality might provide important guidance for U.S. occupational therapists.

The survey was composed of 24 questions. Fifteen questions listed multiple choice responses, and 11 questions were multiple choice for demographics, or short-answer questions to permit optimal expression of respondents' opinions. To minimize bias due to ambiguous terminology, the key terms (spirituality, religion, extrinsic religious life, and intrinsic religious life) were defined by the author and stated on the survey, and respondents were asked to answer the survey questions using the definitions provided (see Appendix A).

Furthermore, the author was interested in sharing clinical tools relevant to problems therapists may be experiencing with the highly subjective and controversial aspects of client spirituality and religion in clinical practice. At the end of the survey, respondents were asked if they wished further information. A list of bibliographic references (detailed in Appendix B) was mailed to respondents who requested further information. Table 9 lists the frequency with which each reference was requested.

The data was analyzed by descriptive analysis to determine frequency of responses. The researcher converted short answer and open ended survey responses via content analysis into quantitative data. A postori coding guided data recording of responses that asked for respondents' comments. The author recorded all original comments provided by respondents while insuring confidentiality. Comments were categorized and described according to content analysis by similar themes. Calculating weighted percent of responses and weighted percent of cases eliminated bias due to uneven size of membership between AOTA and CAOT groups. Weighted percentages were computed based on the percentage of responses made to each separate question.

RESULTS

Thirty-nine percent of Canadian subjects and 38% of U.S. subjects responded to the survey. Insufficient postage was inadvertently provided for the return of surveys from Canadian respondents, which may have decreased the Canadian response rate. A follow-up was not done due to cost and time constraints. Survey results are detailed in Tables 2-9.

A summary of survey results detailed by country is presented in Tables 1-9. For the most part, Canadian and U.S. findings were similar. Due to these similarities and to the large quantity of data obtained, results are discussed here for all respondents, U.S. and Canadian combined.

A brief summary of demographics reveals the mean age of respondents was 37, and 73% had a bachelor's degree. Seventy-five percent of all respondents were full time occupational therapists with a mean of 11 years of experience. One third worked in rehabilitation settings. Forty-nine percent of all respondents worked with clients between 19 and 64 years old. For detailed demographic information, please refer to Table 1. Sixty-three percent of all respondents use eclectic frames of reference (see Table 2 for more information).

Eighty-eight percent of all respondents stated the client's spirituality should be incorporated into practice, while 11% felt occupational therapy should not address the client's spirituality. Spirituality was addressed by 14.5% of all respondents only when the client mentioned it.

TABLE 1. Demographics

Age of Respondent	Mean: 37 years	Median: 35 years	Youngest: 22 years	Eldest: 66 years
Years of Experience	Mean: 11 year	Median: 10 years	Least: 0.25 year	Most: 40 years

Highest Degree Earned	All	Canada	US
Bachelor's Degree in OT	73.2 (443)	79.5 (58)	72.4 (55)
Master's Degree	18 (109)	5.5 (4)	19.7 (15)
Diploma or Certificate in OT	5.1 (31)	13.7 (10)	3.9 (3)
Doctoral Degree	3.6 (22)	1.4 (1)	3.9 (3)
Total responses	100 (605)	100 (73)	100 (76)
Employment Status			
Full-time	74.6 (469)	82.9 (63)	73.4 (58)
Part-time	27.8 (175)	18.4 (14)	29.1 (23)
Setting			
Rehabilitation	33.7 (206)	32.9 (24)	33.8 (26)
Long Term Care	25.2 (154)	19.2 (14)	26 (20)
Acute Care	20.9 (128)	31.5 (23)	19.5 (15)
School	19.8 (121)	12.3 (9)	20.8 (16)
Home Care	12.9 (79)	12.3 (9)	13 (10)
Pediatrics	6.2 (38)	4.1 (3)	6.5 (5)
OT Faculty, Outpatient	5.7 (35)	0	6.5 (5)
Mental Health	5.2 (32)	5.5 (4)	5.2 (4)
Hand Therapy	3.6 (22)	1.4 (1)	3.9 (3)
Rehabilitation	3.4 (21)	0	3.9 (3)
Private Practice	3.1 (19)	6.8 (5)	2.6 (2)
University, Vocational, or Industrial Rehab	2.5 (15)	1.4 (1)	2.6 (2)
AOTF Staff, Subacute	2.3 (14)	0	2.6 (2)
Day Treatment, Development-al Delay, Chronic, Independ-ent Living Center	1.3 (8)	1.4 (1)	1.3 (1)
Community Care	1 (6)	8.2 (6)	0
Geriatrics	0.3 (2)	2.7 (2)	0
Veterans	0.2 (1)	1.4 (1)	0
Total Responses	**(989)**	**(107)**	**(126)**
Professional Duties			
Treat clients on a regular basis	89.8 (510)	87.3 (62)	90.1 (64)
Decide departmental treatment policies	32.7 (186)	35.2 (25)	32.4 (23)
Supervise occupational therapists	30.3 (172)	25.4 (18)	31 (22)
Clients' Age			
Adult (19-64 years)	48.9 (271)	46.5 (33)	49.3 (34)
Older Adult (65+ years)	44.6 (247)	42.3 (30)	44.9 (31)
Children (aged 0-18 years)	33.9 (188)	28.2 (20)	34.8 (24)
Total responses	**(706)**	**(83)**	**(89)**

Note. % (n)

TABLE 2. Respondent's Frames of Reference

	All	**Canada**	**U.S.**
Eclectic frames of reference	63 (358)	60.6 (43)	63.4 (45)
Sensory Integration	7.7 (44)	2.8 (2)	8.5 (6)
Developmental	5.1 (29)	1.4 (1)	5.6 (4)
MOHO	4 (23)	2.8 (2)	4.2 (3)
NDT	2.6 (15)	1.4 (1)	2.8 (2)
Rehabilitation	1.6 (9)	2.8 (2)	1.4 (1)
Occupational Performance	1.4 (8)	11.3 (8)	0
Other	1.4 (8) or less	1.4 (1) or less	1.4 (1) or less
Total responses	**(1396)**	**(171)**	**(192)**

Note. % (n)

Religious affiliation is being assessed by about half of all respondents, 29.8% during chart review or evaluation, 21.9% when the client mentions religion, and 19.4% during treatment. The client's religious affiliation is not being asked by 44.5% of all respondents. Religious affiliation is being used in treatment planning by 84.9% of all respondents; 11.3% of all respondents use the client's religious affiliation to seek social support from the client's faith. Religious affiliation information is not used by 8.9% of all respondents. Six and one-half percent of all respondents report using religious affiliation to refer to clergy for group therapy, and 5.5% of all respondents refer to clergy upon client request. See Table 3 for additional findings.

Concerning whether the client's religion should be addressed in practice, 35.3% of all respondents felt the client's religion should be addressed, and 23% were opposed. Of all respondents, 88.1% felt spirituality was appropriate concern for occupational therapists. (See Table 4 for details.) Fifty-eight percent of all respondents reported having already incorporated spirituality into practice, and 32% have not. Forty-three percent of all respondents have addressed the client's religious life, and 53% have not. See Table 5 for reasons respondents had not addressed the client's spirituality or religion in occupational therapy practice. A majority of all respondents (91%) who are addressing spirituality in practice report using intrinsic activities such as recommending holistic practices; for example, diet, relaxation, Alcoholics Anonymous, or therapeutic touch. Respondents report addressing spirituality with activities to increase self-esteem and locus of control, creating a safe, non-judgmental therapeutic alliance encouraging the client to honestly express feelings, and using activities or rewards which motivate the cli-

TABLE 3. Religious Affiliation Assessment and Use

	All	Canada	U.S.
Religious Affiliation Assessed	47.6 (289)	58.7 (44)	46.1 (35)
During chart review or evaluation	29.8 (181)	36 (27)	28.9 (22)
Only when client mentions it	21.9 (133)	18.7 (14)	22.4 (17)
During treatment	19.4 (118)	26.7 (20)	18.4 (14)
Most clients are asked	15.3 (93)	30.7 (23)	13.2 (10)
Occasionally	13.2 (80)	13.3 (10)	13.2 (10)
Not assessed	44.5 (270)	33.3 (25)	46.1 (35)
Total responses	**(1164)**	**(163)**	**(143)**
Religious Affiliation Used:			
For treatment planning	84.9 (248)	80.9 (38)	85.7 (30)
Involve social support from client's faith	11.3 (33)	10.6 (5)	11.4 (4)
Not used	8.9 (26)	10.6 (5)	8.6 (3)
Refer to clergy for appropriate group therapy	6.5 (19)	10.6 (5)	5.7 (2)
Refer to clergy upon client's request	5.5 (16)	4.3 (2)	5.7 (2)
Total responses	**(342)**	**(55)**	**(41)**

Note. % (n)

ent as a vehicle for achieving goals. Respondents also report spirituality is being addressed by discussing hope and purpose in life related to goal setting. Table 8 lists additional ideas for addressing spirituality.

Seventy-eight percent of all respondents who address religion use extrinsic religious activities such as functional ability to participate in worship, Bible study groups, prayer groups, religious holidays, referrals to clergy, and church accessibility issues (Canada, 88.9%; U.S., 75.8%). In addition, 73% of all respondents incorporate intrinsic religious activity into occupational therapy, such as developing positive coping skills by encouraging hope, faith, and prayer.

Respondents report incorporating spirituality into practice while focusing on anxiety and stress management, social skills training, communication skills, expressing feelings, assertiveness training, life skills training, and engaging parents in the child's therapy. Respondents report involving spirituality in activities of daily living such as dressing for worship and knitting a gift for a baby (an altruistic activity as well hand dexterity therapy).

TABLE 4. Summary of Spirituality and Religion Relative to Practice

	All	Canada	U.S.
Occupational therapists should address spirituality.	88.1 (526)	98.6 (71)	86.7 (65)
Occupational therapists should address religion.	35.3 (211)	50 (36)	33.3 (25)
Occupational therapists should not address religion.	22.6 (135)	12.5 (9)	24 (18)
Occupational therapists should not address spirituality.	10.6 (63)	0	12 (9)
Total responses	**(935)**	**(116)**	**(117)**

Note. % (n)

TABLE 5. Reasons Respondents Had Not Addressed Spirituality or Religion

	All	Canada	U.S.
Not relevant to setting	34.4 (94)	28.6 (10)	35.3 (12)
Not trained to address client's religious life	31.1 (85)	42.9 (15)	29.4 (10)
Client is not capable of addressing these issues due to diagnosis, or client is too young	27.1 (74)	11.4 (4)	29.4 (10)
No right to ask, too personal	23.1 (63)	20 (7)	23.5 (8)
Not trained to address spirituality	12.8 (35)	20 (7)	11.8 (4)
Client hasn't mentioned it	12.1 (33)	14.3 (5)	11.8 (4)
Therapist not comfortable with own spirituality or religious life	5.9 (16)	5.7 (2)	5.9 (2)
Not enough time	5.9 (16)	5.7 (2)	5.9 (2)
Third party payers may not reimburse	2.6 (7)	0	2.9 (1)
Supervisor doesn't support addressing spirituality or religious life	2.6 (7)	0	2.9 (1)
Total responses	**(437)**	**(52)**	**(55)**

Note. % (n)

DISCUSSION

The results of this survey are generally supported by other research on spirituality and religion. Occupational therapists feel that addressing spirit and religion is appropriate for occupational practice, and methodologies are being refined. The results provide additional information to the body of knowledge in that specific information of interest to practitioners is identified.

Many respondents were concerned with how to objectively address spirituality without the imposing the therapist's belief systems. Guidelines developed by the American Psychological Association (APA), from the nursing profession, as well as research from the study of reli-

TABLE 6. Respondents' Difficulties Addressing Spirituality

	All	Canada	U.S.
Procedural issues (i.e. whether to discuss spirituality, assessment, and application to treatment).	74.3 (251)	80.4 (41)	73.2 (30)
Guidance needed	40.2 (136)	60.8 (31)	36.6 (22)
Third party payers won't reimburse	10.7 (36)	2 (1)	12.2 (5)
Not appropriate for an occupational therapist to discuss	8.9 (30)	3.9 (2)	9.8 (4)
Not enough time	7.1 (24)	5.9 (3)	7.3 (3)
Not supported by supervisor	6.5 (22)	2 (1)	7.3 (3)
Not supported by facility; Family may object	5 (17)	5.9 (3)	4.9 (2)
Not supported by team member; therefore, refers to clergy	3.6 (12)	9.8 (5)	2.4 (1)
Not comfortable discussing spirituality	2.4 (8)	2 (1)	2.4 (1)
Total responses	**(553)**	**(91)**	**(66)**

Note. % (n)

TABLE 7. Respondents' Difficulties Addressing Religion

	All	Canada	U.S.
Guidance needed regarding professional boundaries	58.1 (222)	41.3 (19)	60.4 (20)
Procedural issues (i.e., whether to discuss religion, assessing religion, application to treatment, unaware of client's religious practices)	55 (210)	60.9 (28)	54.2 (26)
Not appropriate for an occupational therapist to discuss religion (i.e., due to client's diagnosis, or religion hasn't come up)	31.9 (122)	21.7 (10)	33.3 (16)
Not supported by a team member; refer the client to clergy	14.1 (54)	10.9 (5)	14.6 (7)
Not enough time to address religion	6.3 (24)	6.5 (3)	6.3 (3)
Third party payer may not reimburse	3.7 (14)	0	4.2 (2)
Client's family might object	4.5 (17)	6.5 (3)	4.2 (2)
Other	2.6 (10)	6.5 (3)	2.1 (1)
Not comfortable discussing religion	1 (4)	8.7 (4)	0
Not supported by supervisor	0.3 (1)	2.2 (1)	0
Not supported by facility	0.8 (3)	6.5 (3)	0
Total responses	**(681)**	**(79)**	**(86)**

Note. % (n)

gion may be appropriate for occupational therapy practice. The APA (1990) has issued official guidelines by which psychiatrists may avoid conflict between their own religious convictions and those of the client. Generally, the guidelines stipulate that the psychiatrist should respect the patient's beliefs by learning the tenets of the patient's faith, thereby

TABLE 8. Respondents' Suggested Methods to Address Spirituality

	All	Canada	U.S.
Therapist encourages the client to identify and pursue own goals	62.1 (284)	79.3 (46)	59.6 (34)
Client is encouraged to identify one's own interests	60.4 (276)	77.6 (45)	57.9 (33)
Therapist uses activities to increase client's self-esteem	40 (183)	37.9 (22)	40.4 (23)
Client improves communication with significant other	39.6 (181)	46.6 (27)	38.6 (22)
Client express feelings nonverbally	37.2 (170)	27.6 (16)	38.6 (22)
Client acknowledges one's own strengths	35 (160)	34.5 (20)	35.1 (20)
Client acknowledges one's own weaknesses	30.6 (140)	36.2 (21)	29.8 (17)
Therapist teaches the client stress management techniques	27.4 (125)	22.4 (13)	28.1 (16)
Client does an altruistic activity	16.4 (75)	8.6 (5)	17.5 (10)
Client expresses spirituality in activities of daily living	9.2 (42)	12.1 (7)	8.8 (5)
Client does a self-nurturing activity	7.9 (36)	1.7 (1)	5.3 (3)
Client does an activity involving nature or animals	5 (23)	3.4 (2)	5.3 (3)
Client identifies and reads non-religious motivational literature	4.8 (22)	1.7 (1)	5.3 (3)
Client does an exercise program	3.7 (17)	5.2 (3)	3.5 (2)
Client watches motivational movie or broadcast	0.2 (1)	1.7 (1)	0
Total responses	**(1735)**	**(230)**	**(215)**

Note. % (n)

enabling the psychiatrist to attend to therapeutic needs. The clinician must not impose religious beliefs or ideological systems onto the patient, nor suggest that the patient reinterpret religious convictions in terms of psychological concepts. Rosenfeld (2000) supports this ethical approach for occupational therapists addressing the client's religious life, emphasizing "it is the patient's spirituality that is relevant, and not [the therapist's]" (p. 19).

The researcher expected to find a larger number of Canadian occupational therapists utilizing this frame of reference. Eleven and three-tenths percent of respondents reported using the occupational performance frame of reference, as recommended in the *Occupational Therapy Guidelines for Client-Centred Practice* (CAOT, 1991). The results of this survey indicate that nearly all of the Canadian respondents feel that spirituality is appropriate for occupational therapy practice, an increase of about 50% from Blain and Townsend's survey in 1993. This research also reinforces Blain and Townsend's findings that the majority of Canadian occupational therapists are not sure how to implement spirituality into practice, particularly regarding boundaries and ethical issues.

TABLE 9. Bibliographic Information Requested

	All	Canada	U.S.
A frame of reference incorporating spirituality	57.6 (235)	55.2 (32)	58 (29)
Ideas for incorporating spirituality into treatment planning	59.8 (244)	82.8 (48)	56 (28)
Occupational therapy intervention for spiritual crisis	48.5 (198)	63.8 (37)	46 (23)
An assessment of morale (agitation, attitude on own aging, loneliness, dissatisfied with life)	46.8 (191)	51.7 (30)	46 (23)
A theoretical concept to assess spiritual wellness	47.1 (192)	65.5 (38)	44 (22)
An assessment for spiritual crisis	45.3 (185)	53.4 (31)	44 (22)
Ideas to incorporate religion into treatment planning	38 (155)	50 (29)	36 (18)
Classifying the role of religion in the client's life	26.2 (107)	27.6 (16)	26 (13)
Maintaining professional boundaries with the client's religious life	19.9 (81)	31 (18)	18 (9)
Validated assessment of commitment to religious affiliation	18.9 (77)	24.1 (14)	18 (9)
Total responses	**(1665)**	**(293)**	**(196)**

Note. % (n)

Many of the survey respondents identified practical ways in which they have incorporated clients' spirituality or religion into practice. For instance, respondents are using the Bible for page turning dexterity activities, and respondents suggest that clients resume reading religious literature as a stress reduction strategy. Another respondent provides Native American spirituality support for a terminally ill Native American. Another therapist described discussing issues of hope and purpose in life relating to goal-setting and future orientation with suicidal patients. Also, a respondent suggests reminding the client that it is appropriate to ask for help when the client is not able to complete a task. A respondent recommended helping the client identify a *raison d'être*, and acknowledge the client's personal successes. These recommendations are consistent with Carpenito's suggestions for nurses addressing spiritual distress (1993).

This study replicated many of the findings published by Taylor et al. (2000). Specifically, the majority of Taylor et al.'s respondents agreed that spirituality is a fundamental aspect of being human; one's spirituality influences his or her health, that disease and disability affect clients' spirituality and that knowledge of spiritual beliefs and practices is essential for occupational therapy practice. Furthermore, most of these respondents agreed holistic treatment should include the mind, body, and spirit, not just the mind and body.

SHOULD OCCUPATIONAL THERAPISTS ADDRESS SPIRITUALITY OR RELIGION?

A client's spiritual and religious life is appropriate for occupational therapy practice for a variety of reasons. Ethically, an occupational therapist has a fiduciary relationship with the client (Moyers, 2000). Therefore, by definition, occupational therapists must design treatment plans that are relevant to the client's culture, values, morals, and priorities. In short, occupational therapists are obligated to develop treatment plans that are meaningful to the patient and engage or motivate the patient's spirit.

In addition, healing is enhanced when the client is practicing his or her chosen religion on a personal level (Koenig, Kvale, & Ferrel, 1988; Koenig, 1995; Wirth, 1993). Designing meaningful therapeutic activities is done effectively by addressing values which motivate the client's spirit, thereby enhancing the possibility of return to independence (Urbanowski & Vargo, 1994).

In her work with persons with acquired immune deficiency syndrome (AIDS), Gutterman (1990) found that "spirituality and occupational therapy interconnect when we define spirit as the life source within us that tells us who we really are. Occupational therapists can stimulate, or inspire, the client toward self-actualization and insight by teaching or providing opportunities for learning self-healing techniques" (p. 236). One of the essential reasons we develop therapeutic goals with our clients is to validate and reinforce lifestyle patterns that promote and sustain long term wellness. Addressing the client's spirit means to understand the client's values, what he or she feels is meaningful, and what stirs the client to be active. This requires interactive clinical reasoning skills such as active listening, authenticity, nonjudgmental observation, perceiving the client's "story" (Mattingly & Fleming, 1994), and therapeutic use of self. The clinician develops rapport with the client by addressing his or her spirit with a sense of caring and by communicating with an attitude of unconditional acceptance. Rapport continues to develop as the clinician honestly communicates in a style that the client can absorb and understand. Most of these strategies do not require extra treatment time, but rather effective communication and clinical reasoning. The author has found these strategies have worked with clients who present for treatment with apparently little interest in complying with therapy of any kind.

In today's reimbursement-driven environment, occupational therapists must efficiently utilize all resources to shorten the course of treatment without compromising outcome. By reinforcing religious practice on a personal level, the occupational therapist may quickly forge a meaningful therapeutic alliance and increase potential for long-term wellness. Congregations and religious professionals may offer powerful support networks to facilitate discharge planning, enhance community reintegration, and optimize outcome.

Assessment

The client's spirituality and religious life is perceived by CAOT as the basis for meaningful occupational therapy intervention (1991). Egan and DeLaat (1994) conceptualize spirit as the most basic performance area in occupational therapy upon which the client is motivated to function in daily activity. Review of religious journals provides a paradigm of assessment of spiritual wellness which may be helpful as a clinical reasoning scheme to assess the client's views separate from the therapist's religious or spiritual values.

In working with a client's spirituality or religious life, an objective assessment of the client's spiritual wellness needs to be made. Chandler, Holden, and Kolander (1992) developed a model for assessing spiritual wellness, which may prove to be a valuable clinical reasoning tool for objective assessment. The central theme of this model relies on assessing balance in the subject's life. Chandler et al. (1992) describe "balance as two dimensions of spiritual wellness: repression of the sublime at one end of the horizontal continuum, and spiritual emergency (preoccupation with spirituality to the detriment of wellness) at the other end. On the vertical axis, "one may demonstrate any stage along a continuum of spiritual development" (p. 170). Spiritual development can be assessed indirectly by interviewing the person concerning his or her personal development (age, maturation level), and degree of health with that stage of development (level of emotional, occupational, physical, intellectual, and social functioning). Spiritual wellness is perceived as a balance between alienating oneself from the world versus involvement with one's spirituality to the exclusion of the rest of the world. The authors recommend therapeutic interventions such as meditation and creative visualization to achieve balance between these extremes as chaotic events (i.e., resulting in illness or grief) challenge spiritual wellness and growth.

Rapport

Carpenito (1993) has developed a model for addressing religion and spirituality in nursing practice. She noted that our clients who are most prone to spiritual distress include those who have a terminal illness, loss of a body part, chronic pain, trauma, miscarriage, abortion, surgery, dietary restrictions, isolation, death of a significant other, lack of privacy, or lack of support for one's chosen faith perspective. Carpenito suggests an approach for discussing and meeting the client's religious and spiritual needs which is compatible with the SOAP note writing style. This model seems germane for many patients that occupational therapists and nurses treat. *Subjective Data:* Ask the client whether he or she is religious. Ask the client what he or she does to reduce stress or find a source of strength. *Objective Data:* Does the patient present with signs and symptoms of stress, depression, or spiritual crisis? Who is the client's religious leader? Have the client's religious convictions or practices changed recently? Is the client preoccupied with resolving spiritual concerns? Is the client satisfied with his ability to fulfill chosen roles? (1993, p. 747).

Carpenito (1993) also has suggested ways of interacting with the client:

- ask the client's priorities,
- actively listen to the client; talk with the client, not to the client,
- create a mood of unconditional positive regard with the client,
- encourage the client to express his or her feelings,
- ask the client in what circumstances he or she has felt fulfilled, worthy, and valued,
- respect cultural and religious diversity,
- support the expression of client's cultural and spiritual needs,
- provide ways for the facility or family to provide ethnic foods,
- create opportunities for client privacy and personal time, and
- ask the client how to help meet his or her religious or spiritual needs.

LIMITATIONS

This survey is a pilot study and the survey instrument was not validated or rated for reliability. Respondents did not necessarily answer all survey questions, possibly due to survey length, redundant questions, or the sensitivity of the material. Also, the Canadian response rate may have been limited by incorrect postage on the return.

RECOMMENDATIONS

Given the respondents' ambivalence and expressed need for more training in addressing spirituality and religion in occupational therapy practice, the author offers the following recommendations. Spirituality course work should be developed in occupational therapy schools and for continuing education workshops. More than 34 medical schools in the United States are incorporating spirituality training or alternative medicine into curriculum (Shapiro, 1997; Behar, 1997), a reflection of the public's interest in these topics and medicine's growing awareness of the relevance for optimum health care. Perhaps the findings of this study may help occupational therapists in the U.S. and Canada refine strategies for addressing the client's spirituality or religious life effectively in occupational therapy practice.

CONCLUSION

Developing truly meaningful treatment plans for an individual client requires the occupational therapist to perceive the client's cultural values, spiritual motivations, and religious practice. In so doing, the therapist may improve therapeutic rapport, treatment compliance, and improve outcomes by utilizing the mind-body connection to optimize healing and return to function. Many respondents appear willing to address the client's spiritual and religious life, and would like professional training in this regard.

ACKNOWLEDGMENTS

Thanks to Bill Moyers for producing the inspirational video *Healing and the Mind,* to Michael Pizzi, MS, OTR/L, CHES, to the occupational therapists at *Youville Hospital and Rehabilitation Center,* Cambridge, MA,. The author is grateful for the assistance of Helen Smith, MOT, OTR, FAOTA, Diana M. Bailey, EdD, OTR, FAOTA, and Ann McClintock, OTR, who provided the support necessary for completion of this project. Special thanks are extended to Jodi Carlson for her editorial support. This research was funded by the American Occupational Therapy Foundation.

REFERENCES

American Occupational Therapy Association. (2000, July). American Occupational Therapy Association Standards of Practice [Internet]. *<http://www.aota.org/otsp. asp>* Preface.

American Psychiatric Association. (1994). *Diagnostic and statistical manual of mental disorders* (4th ed.). Washington, DC: Author.

American Psychological Association. (1990). Guidelines regarding possible conflict between psychiatrists' religious commitments and psychiatric practice. *American Journal of Psychiatry, 147* (4), 542.

Anderson, R. C. (1994). Defining rehabilitation chaplaincy as a specialty within pastoral care. *Journal of Religion in Disability & Rehabilitation, 1*(1), 53-68.

Behar, M. (1997). Reiki: Bridging traditional and complementary healing techniques. *OT Practice,* February, 22-23.

Benson, H. & Klipper, M. Z. (1975). *The relaxation response.* New York: Avon Books.

Benson, H. & Proctor, W. (1985). *Beyond the relaxation response.* New York: Berkley Books.

Benson, H. & Proctor, W. (1987). *Your maximum mind.* New York: Avon Books.

Benson, H. (1996, December). *Introduction.* Paper presented at the conference entitled "Spirituality & Healing in Medicine-II," Boston.

Blain, J. & Townsend, E. (1993). Occupational therapy guidelines for client-centred practice: Impact study findings. *Canadian Journal of Occupational Therapy,* December, *60*(5), 271-285.

Brown, L. B. (1964). Classifications of religious orientation. *Journal for the Scientific Study of Religion, 4,* 91-99.

Burkhardt, A. (1997). Occupational therapy & wellness. *OT Practice,* June, 28-35.

Burnard, P. (1988). Discussing spiritual issues with clients. *Health Visitor, 61,* 371-372.

Canadian Association of Occupational Therapists. (1991). *Occupational therapy guidelines for client-centred practice.* Author: Toronto.

Carpenito, L. J. (1993). *Nursing diagnosis: Application to clinical practice* (5th ed.). Philadelphia: J. B. Lippincott Company.

Chandler, C. K., Holden, J. M., & Kolander, C. A. (1992). Counseling for spiritual wellness: Theory and practice. *Journal of Counseling and Development, 71,* 168-175.

Colgrove, M., Bloomfield, H., & McWilliams, P. (1991). *How to survive the loss of a love.* Los Angeles: Prelude Press.

Cousins, N. (1989). Belief becomes biology. *Advances, 6*(3), 20-29.

Dombeck, M., & Karl, J. (1987). Spiritual issues in mental health care. *Journal of Religion and Health, 26* (3), 183-197.

Egan, M. & DeLaat, M. D. (1994). Considering spirituality in occupational therapy practice. *Canadian Journal of Occupational Therapy, 61*(2), 95-101.

Engquist, D., Short-DeGraff, M., Gliner, J., & Oltjenbruns, K. (1997). Occupational therapists' beliefs and practices with regard to spirituality and therapy. *The American Journal of Occupational Therapy, 51 (3), 173-180.*

Giglio, J. (1993). The impact of patients' and therapists' religious values on psychotherapy. *Hospital and Community Psychiatry, 44*(8), 768-771.

Gutterman, L. (1990). A day treatment program for persons with AIDS. *American Journal of Occupational Therapy, 44*(3), 234-237.

Hoge, D. R. (1972). A validated intrinsic religious motivation scale. *Journal for the Scientific Study of Religion, 11,* 369-376.

Kabat-Zinn, J. (1990). *Full catastrophe living: Using the wisdom of your body and mind to face stress, pain, and illness.* New York: Dell Publishing.

Koenig, H. G. (1994). *Aging and God: Spiritual pathways to mental health in midlife and later years.* New York: The Haworth Press, Inc.

Koenig, H. G. (1995). *Research on religion and aging: An annotated bibliography.* Westport, CT: Greenwood Publishing Group, Inc.

Koenig, H. G., Kvale, J. N., & Ferrel, C. (1988). Religion and well being in later life. *The Gerontologist, 28*(1), 18-28.

Lawton, M. P. (1975). The Philadelphia Geriatric Center Morale Scale: A revision. *Journal of Gerontology, 30* (1), 85-89.

Magida, A. J., (Ed.) (1996). *How to be a perfect stranger: A guide to etiquette in other people's religious ceremonies.* Woodstock, VT: Jewish Lights Publishing.

Mattingly, C. & Fleming, M. (1994). *Clinical reasoning: Forms of inquiry in a therapeutic practice.* Philadelphia: F. A. Davis Company.

McColl, M. A. (1994). Holistic occupational therapy: Historical meanings and contemporary implications. *Canadian Journal of Occupational Therapy, 61* (2), 72-77.

McCormack, G. L. (1992). Psychoneuroimmunology: A model for occupational therapy. *Occupational Therapy Practice, 3*(4), 1-11.

Melnechuk, T. (1988). Emotions, brain, immunity, and health: A review. In M. Clynes & J. Panksepp (Eds.) *Emotions and psychopathology.* New York: Plenum Press.

Miller, J. S. (1990). Mental illness and spiritual crisis: Implications for psychiatric rehabilitation. *Psychosocial Rehabilitation Journal, 14* (2), 29-47.

Moyers, B., Flowers, B. S., & Grubin, D. (Eds.) (1993). *Healing and the mind.* New York: Doubleday.

Moyers, P. (2000, May). *Best practice: The guide to occupational therapy.* Vermont Occupational Therapy Association 2000 Annual Conference, White River Junction, Vermont.

Muldoon, M. & King, J. N. (1991). A spirituality for the long haul: Response to chronic illness. *Journal of Religion and Health, 30*(2), 99-108.

Oleckno, W. A. & Blacconiere, M. J. (1991). Relationship of religiosity to wellness and other health-related behaviors and outcomes. *Psychological Reports, 68,* 819-826.

Perr, A. (1994). Adaptive equipment: Freedom and independence for people with disabilities. *Journal of Religion in Disability & Rehabilitation, 1*(1), 81-87.

Pert, C. (1993). The chemical communicators. In B. Moyers, B. S. Flowers, and D. Grubin (Eds.), *Healing and the mind* (pp. 177-194). New York: Doubleday.

Quiroga, V. (1995). *Occupational therapy: The first 30 years: 1900-1930.* Bethesda, MD: The American Occupational Therapy Association, Inc.

Rosenfeld, M. S. (2000). Spiritual agent modalities for occupational therapy practice. *OT Practice,* January, 17-21.

Salewski, R. M. (1993). Meeting holistic health needs through a religious organization: The congregation. *Journal of Holistic Nursing, 11*(2), 183-196.

Shapiro, E. (1997). Spirituality speeds recovery of patients. *The Medical Herald,* May, p. 38.

Stahl, C. (1994). Has OT found a model for spiritual evaluation? *Advance for Occupational Therapists,* October 24, 1994: *10*(42), p. 5, 20.

Taylor, E., Mitchell, J. E., Kenan, S, & Tacker, R. (2000). Attitudes of occupational therapists toward spirituality in practice. *American Journal of Occupational Therapy Association, 54,* 421-426.

Urbanowski, R. & Vargo, J. (1994). Spirituality, daily practice, and the occupational performance model. *Canadian Journal of Occupational Therapy, 61*(2), 88-94.

Urbanowski, R. (1997, December). Spirituality in everyday practice. *Occupational Therapy Practice, 2*(12), 18-23.

Whyte, N. (1997). T'ai Chi for clients in cardiac rehabilitation. *Occupational Therapy Practice, 2*(10), 38-41.

Wirth, D. P. (1993). Implementing spiritual healing in modern medical practice. *Advances, the Journal of Mind-Body Health, 9*(4), 69-81.

APPENDIX A. Definitions in Survey Instrument

Spirituality

that emotional and volitional energy which animates a person, the source by which the client derives meaning in everyday life. Spirituality may exist within the client independent of the presence of religious beliefs and practices. Examples of spirituality in occupational therapy practice include improving communication with a significant other, expressing one's feelings, respecting one's own needs, performing altruistic activities, and unconditional positive regard for another's views (Chandler, Holden, & Kolander, 1992; Dombeck, 1994; Urbanowski & Vargo, 1994).

Religion

"an organized body of thought and experience concerning the fundamental problems of existence; an organized system of faith" (Dombeck, 1994, p. 184).

Extrinsic religious life

includes "group religious activities such as attending worship services, Bible study groups, prayer groups, adult religious classes offered by the client's religious organization, church or synagogue social gatherings" (Koenig, Kvale, & Ferrel, 1988, p. 21).

Intrinsic religious life

"activities the client can do alone, such as reading the Bible or other religious doctrines, reading religious magazines and literature, watching religious television programs, watching religious movies, or listening to religious radio broadcasts" (Koenig, Kvale, & Ferrel, 1988, p. 21)

APPENDIX B. Resources for Addressing Religion and Spirituality

maintaining professional boundaries	American Psychological Association (1990); Giglio, J. (1993); and Rosenfeld, M. S. (2000).
theoretical concept to assess spiritual wellness	Chandler, C., Holden, J., & Kolander, C. (1992); Stahl, C. (1994).
an assessment for spiritual crisis	American Psychiatric Association. (1994); Chandler, C. K., Holden, J. M., & Kolander, C. A. (1992).
intervention for spiritual crisis	Behar, M. (1997); Gutterman, L. (1990); Miller, J. S. (1990).
assessment of morale	Lawton, M. P. (1975).
validated assessment for commitment to religious life	Hoge, D. R. (1972).
classifying the role of religion	Brown, L. B. (1964).
frame of reference which includes spirituality	Blain, J. & Townsend, E. (1993); Canadian Association of Occupational Therapists (1991); Egan, M. & DeLaat, M. D. (1994); Urbanowski, R. & Vargo, J. (1994).
incorporating spirituality into treatment planning	Burnard, P. (1988); Behar, M. (1997); Bellert, J. L. (1989); Canadian Association of Occupational Therapists (1991); Colgrove, M., Bloomfield, H. H., & McWilliams, P. (1991); Miller, J. S. (1990); Perry, J. W. (1986); Stahl, C. (Ed.) (1993); Urbanowski, R. & Vargo, J. (1994); Wirth, D. P. (1993).

Index

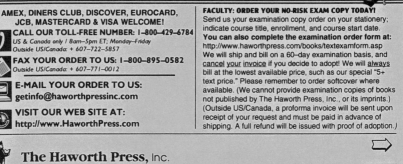

TO ORDER: CALL: 1-800-429-6784 / FAX: 1-800-895-0582 (Outside US/Canada: + 607-771-0012) / E-MAIL: getinfo@haworthpressinc.com

☐ YES, please send me **Caregiving—Leisure and Aging**

___ in hard at $39.95 ISBN: 0-7890-0776-2.

___ in soft at $19.95 ISBN: 0-7890-0799-1.

- Individual orders outside US, Canada, and Mexico must be prepaid by check or credit card.
- Discounts are not available on 5+ text prices and not available in conjunction with any other discount. • Discount not applicable on books priced under $15.00.
- Postage & handling: In US: $4.00 for first book & $1.50 for each additional book. Outside US: $5.00 for first book; $2.00 for each additional book.
- Canadian residents: please add appropriate sales tax after postage & handling. Canadian residents: please add 7% GST after postage & handling. Canadian residents of Newfoundland, Nova Scotia, and New Brunswick, also add 8% for province tax. • Payment in UNESCO coupons welcome.
- If paying in Canadian dollars, use current exchange rate to convert to US dollars.
- Please allow 3–4 weeks for delivery after publication.
- Prices and discounts subject to change without notice.

Signature _____

☐ BILL ME LATER($5 service charge will be added).
(Not available for individuals outside US/Canada/Mexico. Service charge is waived for jobbers/wholesalers/booksellers.)

☐ Check here if billing address is different from shipping address and attach purchase order and billing address information.

☐ PAYMENT ENCLOSED $ _____
(Payment must be in US or Canadian dollars by check or money order drawn on a US or Canadian bank.)

☐ PLEASE BILL MY CREDIT CARD:

☐ AmEx ☐ Diners Club ☐ Discover ☐ Eurocard ☐ JCB ☐ Master Card ☐ Visa

Account Number _____

Expiration Date _____

Signature _____
May we open a confidential credit card account for you for possible future purchases? ( ) Yes ( ) No

Please complete the information below or tape your business card in this area.

NAME _____

INSTITUTION _____

ADDRESS _____

CITY _____

STATE _____ ZIP _____

COUNTRY _____

COUNTY (NY residents only) _____

E-MAIL _____

May we use your e-mail address for confirmations and other types of information? ( ) Yes ( ) No We appreciate receiving your e-mail address and fax number. Haworth would like to e-mail or fax special discount offers to you, as a preferred customer. We will never **share, rent, or exchange** your e-mail address or fax number. We regard such actions as an invasion of your privacy.

☐ YES, please send me **Caregiving—Leisure and Aging (ISBN: 0-7890-0799-1.)** to consider on a 60-day **no risk** examination basis. I understand that I will receive an invoice payable within 60 days, or that **if I decide to adopt the book, my invoice will be cancelled.** I understand that I will be billed at the lowest price. (60-day offer available only to teaching faculty in US, Canada, and Mexico / Outside US/Canada, a proforma invoice will be sent upon receipt of your request and must be paid in advance of shipping. A full refund will be issued with proof of adoption.)

Signature _____

Course Title(s) _____

Current Text(s) _____

Enrollment _____

Semester _____ Decision Date _____

Office Tel _____ Hours _____

This information is needed to process your examination copy order.

FAX

THE HAWORTH PRESS, INC., 10 Alice Street, Binghamton, NY 13904–1580 USA

(06) (19) 10/01 BIC01

FAX